Other Books by Bernard Seeman

The River of Life

Man Against Pain

How to Live with Diabetes (*with Henry Dolger, M.D.*)

YOUR SIGHT:
Folklore, Fact and Common Sense

YOUR SIGHT

FOLKLORE, FACT AND COMMON SENSE

by Bernard Seeman

LITTLE, BROWN and COMPANY

Boston   Toronto

Photographs courtesy *Research to Prevent Blindness, Inc.*

Diagrams courtesy *Alcon Laboratories, Inc.*

Copyright © 1968 BY BERNARD SEEMAN

All rights reserved. No part of this book may be reproduced in any form or by any electronic or mechanical means including information storage and retrieval systems without permission in writing from the publisher, except by a reviewer who may quote brief passages in a review.   Library of Congress Catalog Card No. 68-14740

FIRST EDITION

Published simultaneously in Canada by Little, Brown & Company (Canada) Limited

PRINTED IN THE UNITED STATES OF AMERICA

Acknowledgments

The author makes grateful acknowledgment to the National Society for the Prevention of Blindness, Inc., and to Research to Prevent Blindness, Inc., for information they made available. Of particular value was the scientific material presented at the National Seminar in Ophthalmology conducted in Washington, D.C., under the sponsorship of Research to Prevent Blindness, Inc.

Contents

PART ONE: The Sense of Sight

Chapter 1	The Meaning of Sight	3
Chapter 2	The Development of Sight	7
Chapter 3	The Magic Eye	14
Chapter 4	From the Earliest View	18
Chapter 5	The Seeing Eye	26
Chapter 6	Recognition	46

CONTENTS

PART TWO: The Problems of Sight

Chapter 7	What the Problems Are	57
Chapter 8	Myopia, Hyperopia and Astigmatism	64
Chapter 9	The Aging Eye	67
Chapter 10	Strabismus and Amblyopia: Deviated and Weakened Eyes	72
Chapter 11	Glaucoma	81
Chapter 12	Cataract: A Curtain Against Light	89
Chapter 13	The Detached Retina	98
Chapter 14	Diabetic and Hypertensive Retinopathy	106
Chapter 15	Uveitis: The Inflamed Interior	113
Chapter 16	Vitreous and the Optic Nerve	119
Chapter 17	Hazards to the Eye's Exterior	123
Chapter 18	Tumors and Other Problems	137
Chapter 19	The Sensitive Eye	141

PART THREE: Protecting Your Sight

Chapter 20	Accidents and First Aid	151
Chapter 21	Defending Your Eyes	156
Chapter 22	Protecting Children's Eyes	163

PART FOUR: Aid for Your Eyes

Chapter 23	New Horizons for the Blind and Near-Blind	175
Chapter 24	Eyeglasses	183

CONTENTS

Chapter 25	Contact Lenses	*193*
Chapter 26	Eyes on the Future	*201*
	APPENDIX	*219*
	BIBLIOGRAPHY	*225*
	GLOSSARY	*227*
	INDEX	*237*

THE SENSE OF SIGHT

1

THE SENSE OF SIGHT

1

THE SENSE OF SIGHT

The Meaning of Sight 1

What is sight to us?

Ordinarily we accept it without question and without thought.

Unlikely though it might be, imagine that you wake up one morning and see . . . nothing. You can hear the ticking of the clock but you cannot see the time on its face. You cannot tell whether it is day or night. The sun, if it is shining, is invisible to you.

Then imagine all of the other acts you usually perform each morning upon arising: taking a shower; picking out the toothpaste from the other tubes and brushing your teeth; shaving or making up, along with choosing the right lipstick and other cosmetics;

selecting your clothing for the day, making sure the colors are matched; preparing breakfast; and the thousand and one other details that only begin your average day.

Suddenly, this morning, you must do them in utter darkness: by touch, by sound, by smell, by taste, by memory, but without sight.

Familiar faces will now go unseen — the husband or wife, the child — and new faces will never come into view. There are the familiar sights — the changing colors of the seasons, the starry sweep of the night sky, children at play, the family gathered around the tree at Christmas — none to be seen again.

What is sight to us?

Admittedly, life is possible without sight. There are creatures that have evolved in lightless caverns and in the depths of the ocean abysses, certain fish and lizards that need no sight because theirs is a world of perpetual darkness. They must depend upon other senses, as do the blind among us.

But ours is a universe of light as well as of sound, smell, taste, and texture. Sight is far more than merely a means of perceiving objects. It is, along with our other senses, a shield against danger and a fundamental weapon of survival. On a most primitive level, sight is a means of detecting food and, equally, of avoiding becoming food.

If our early ancestors did not see the saber-toothed tiger, they soon found themselves inside it. This, to a great extent, is the framework within which sight evolved. The creatures that had greater awareness of their environment — of its hazards and its sanctuaries, of which were the eaters and what could be eaten — were able to survive and pass into the future. Those with lesser awareness perished, and their genetic lines were obliterated.

What is sight to us?

Without it, we would have been unable to shape the simplest stone knifeblade or spearhead, make fire, invent the wheel, or send a computerized rocket to the stars. Unable to see, we could never even have entered history, much less come to shape it.

The Nature of Light

The sixteenth-century French poet Guillaume de Salluste du Bartas referred to the eyes as "These lovely lamps, these windows of the soul."

Had he turned outward rather than inward, he might well have said, "These lovely lamps, these windows upon the universe."

We do, literally, perceive the universe through our eyes. Thanks to the electron microscope man can probe the infinitesimal to see the structure of a molecule of matter. And at night he can turn his eyes to the sky and see great galaxies — island universes that dwarf the Milky Way but, because of their unimaginable distances from earth, appear to the naked eye as flickering spots of light.

Actually, we do not see objects. We see neither the molecule of matter nor the galaxy, nor even the page of a book. We see only light: the light *reflected* by the page, or the light *generated* by the star or galaxy. This light is collected by our eyes and focused upon the retinas. There the light is converted into nerve impulses and sent to the brain, where they are interpreted into the images of what we "see" — the galaxy, the molecule, or the page.

The nature of light remains in great part a mystery, despite the fact that scientists have been studying it for hundreds of years. A number of theories have been developed to describe the phenomenon, but the characteristics of light seem so varied under different circumstances that the theories appear to contradict each other.

Light, for instance, appears to have some of the characteristics of waves: the wavelengths of different kinds of light can even be measured. But under other conditions light acts not as a series of

YOUR SIGHT: FOLKLORE, FACT AND COMMON SENSE

waves but as a shower of particles or bundles of energy, called photons.

What is known as light and perceived through the sense of sight is only a small segment of what was labeled as electromagnetic energy by the nineteenth-century Scottish physicist James Clerk Maxwell. Nor is all of this so-called light visible to man. We "see" only the light that ranges from the red at one side of the spectrum to violet at the other. The longer wavelengths of infrared light, which we perceive as heat, and the shorter wavelengths of ultraviolet are invisible to us.

But what man cannot see, other creatures do find visible. Birds, animals, insects, and fish can see as light parts of the electromagnetic spectrum to which humans are blind. In turn, they may be unable to see light that is plain to our eyes. Birds, for example, are able to see infrared frequencies that are invisible to human sight. On the other hand, they cannot see the blue and violet visible to man. Undisturbed by these light frequencies, which are involved in the blurring effect of so-called "distant haze," birds can see distant objects more sharply than we.

As "windows upon the universe," man's eyes are his most important organs of sense. Of all the messages reaching the brain from the world around us, approximately nine out of ten come through the eyes. Hearing, touch, taste, smell, and pain perception each has a vital role in providing man with information about his environment, warning him of danger, directing him toward food, safety, and pleasing sensations. Of all the senses, sight is certainly the most useful, the one most necessary to well-being and development; and, along with the danger sense of pain, most important to survival.

The Development of Sight 2

Sight in its simplest form is the ability to distinguish light from dark. This does not even require an eye as we know it. Plants, with eyeless sight, can turn their faces to the sun, following its passage across the sky; or, like the crocus, open its bloom to light and close it to darkness.

At the other extreme is the most finely developed sight of all — that of the bird, which has such remarkable eyes that, at one hundred yards, it can clearly see a seed of grain that is barely visible to the human eye at less than five feet.

When the first capsule of life formed on this planet an estimated three billion years ago, it was almost certainly able to re-

YOUR SIGHT: FOLKLORE, FACT AND COMMON SENSE

act to light. Had it been unable to do so, it probably would not have survived. This does not mean that the first living cell already had an eye, but like the single-celled amoeba, its entire outer surface may well have been photosensitive and thus able to react to the radiation we see as light. In this respect, it was all "eye."

The development of a separate organ devoted to seeing alone must have taken millions of years of evolution. Today, such an "eye" can be seen in a tiny aquatic creature with the rather euphonious name of *Euglena viridis*.

Euglena is not as pretty as her name, with her whiplike tail and simple opening that serves as a mouth. What does distinguish *Euglena* is the fact that just below the mouth she has a roundish protuberance that is reddish pink in color and sensitive to light. This rosy knob is an eye. *Euglena* is one of the simplest and most primitive forms in which such a specialized organ has been found.

With her single little bump of an eye *Euglena* does not see form or color. Instead, her eye seems able only to detect different intensities of light. It can distinguish light from darkness, bright light from dim. This latter characteristic was demonstrated some years ago in an experiment reported in the *American Scholar* by Thomas H. Shastel. He placed a specimen of *Euglena* into a chamber that had been divided into three connected compartments. One of the compartments was dark, the middle one was in a sort of twilight, and the third was brightly lighted. When *Euglena* was placed in either of the outer compartments — the dark one or the brightly lighted one — she made her way to the twilight section, where she remained. And when placed into the twilight compartment she was content to rest where she was. Clearly, *Euglena* could not only distinguish light from darkness, but seemed to prefer the gentler zone of twilight to either.

There is a vast gap between the simple photosensitivity of the earliest life forms that developed on this planet and the rosy knob that is *Euglena's* specialized eye. But great as this difference may be, it dwindles to nothing when *Euglena*'s primitive eye is compared with the efficient eye of man. Where *Euglena* can detect only different intensities of light, human eyes can follow the flight of a swallow, see the shifting colors of a sunset, and mark the tracery of a snowflake.

The Evolving Eye

Among all living things other than plants the eye is one of the most common organs. A number of creatures, such as snakes, fish, and worms, do not have limbs. Many, such as most mammals, fish, and reptiles, do not have wings. Some lack hearts or lungs; others, stomachs or kidneys. But almost all animals have eyes or something serving their function.

These eyes are by no means similar in the many species that possess them. This is because the eye did not follow a straight line of development. Instead, scientists believe, hundreds of different paths were followed by the evolving eye, with multitudes of variations among the many millions of life forms that have appeared upon this planet.

Certainly all animate things, including plants, share the common ancestry of those first capsules of living matter that could sense the difference between light and darkness. But very early in time they struck out in different directions of visual development. The light-sensitive apparatus of a morning glory, the compound eye of a fly, and the eye of a man each seems to have followed separate evolutionary paths.

The human eye, like those of other vertebrates, probably began its special development in one of the very early forms of fish. Rather than eyes as such, this fish may have had light-sensitive cells in its skin.

As these fish evolved, their front ends, involved in the all-important task of taking in food, began to take on more specialized tasks that increased their food-gathering efficiency. The front end thus became a head in which certain essential sense organs were concentrated. Under the influence of natural selection, eyes gradually developed.

Originally, these primitive eyes may have extended outward as sensitive bubbles of brain tissue, remaining attached to the brain itself by tubes that served as nerves. Since such bubbles would be extremely sensitive to damage, those that were better protected and less vulnerable survived more readily. Under the pressure of time and natural selection, bony ridges gradually developed around them, as well as tough protective sheaths and coverings.

Some of the early vertebrates had several pairs of eyes so that they could see in many directions, forward, sideways, upward, and even backward. In most creatures the lateral-seeing eyes proved themselves more useful than the top-of-head or parietal eye, and consequently survived. Nevertheless, in lampreys and certain lizards a third eye may still be found in working order, while some frogs have what remains of a parietal eye located between their two large eyes. This tiny vestige of a primitive eye may, scientists believe, still retain some sensitivity to light.

As some vertebrates left the seas in which life first evolved and came to live on land, their eyes needed further protection. Eyelids developed and in some creatures, such as snakes and birds, there were third, *nictitating* eyelids in addition to the upper and lower lids. Snakes have eyelids of a tough, transparent material that cannot ordinarily be seen and act in much the same way as storm windows.

In the human eye as it has presently evolved, the original bubble of brain that formed the more primitive eye collapsed and assumed a cuplike shape. This is the retina, a portion of the eye that still remains a part of the brain itself. This process of retina formation can actually be seen in the embryo, which crowds

THE DEVELOPMENT OF SIGHT

millions of years of evolution from cell to human fetus into a period of about a dozen weeks. First there is the brain-bubble eye, then the forward portion of the bubble collapses and forms a cup-shaped structure which becomes the retina of the true eye.

The fact that humans have relatively sharp vision, much sharper than most of our vertebrate cousins, is due mainly to the peculiar structure of the retina. On the retina, at the optic axis of each eye — that is, directly opposite the center of the pupil — there is a small spot called the *fovea*. This spot, crowded with sensitive nerve cells, makes it possible to distinguish fine details. Were we to lack this fovea, as many creatures do, human eyes would still be able to see objects and distinguish between shapes, but they would lack the acuity to read the print on a page or, possibly, to distinguish one face from another. The snake, which has no fovea, does not possess the discriminating vision of man or even fish. However, it is capable of seeing objects as they move.

The lens of the eye, which collects light and focuses it on the retina, is believed to have developed originally in the fish. This was not the only piscene contribution to the developing eye. Fish also provided the vertebrates that evolved from them with the iris, the pupils, and the muscles that contract the lens and focus it for both near and distant vision.

Human eyes and those of apes and monkeys then underwent some additional improvements to provide us with effective daytime and color vision. (Scientists believe that color vision also developed in some of the very early fish and reptiles. If this is so, the characteristic has apparently been bred out of them. The modern-day fish is unable to see color as man does but, as tests suggest, is aware only of varying shades of gray. Fair color vision does exist in some amphibians.)

Human eyes, while not as sharp or efficient as the eyes of a bird, have evolved over some three billion years as instruments eminently suited to serve our needs. Our eyes can scan a distant panorama or study fine details only inches away. They can separate colors, see in both bright light and dim, warn of danger, and delineate the elements of beauty.

When man's eyes attained their present form, his life expectancy was much shorter than it is today. At that point, the human eye was designed to serve men whose lives were vastly more hectic and much briefer than our own. For these early men, the eye could generally offer efficient service throughout their short and precarious lifetimes, which have been estimated to have averaged approximately eighteen years.

But modern man has developed a host of artificial aids for survival — medicines, weapons that protect him from enemies, better nutrition, and the other paraphernalia of civilization. As a consequence, his life outlasts his body's period of maximum efficiency. So the lens of the eye hardens, the ciliary muscles that control focusing weaken, the eye loses its ability to accommodate for changing distances, and eyeglasses or corrective lenses become necessary.

Once, nature prodded man to evolve better eyes by continuously challenging him. Whoever had the sharpest eyes and the swiftest responses was quicker to see and react to the dangers lurking in the dark, and was able to survive and pass his better vision on to his progeny. He who had less acute vision, could not see the hazards or find scarce food, perished, and his progeny dwindled. So, almost inevitably, eyes kept improving.

Today, man has reduced the challenge of natural selection by creating a largely artificial environment. Even the blind are protected. The sharp, quick eye no longer gives its possessor an edge in the survival struggle. Consequently, since even those with defective sight survive and pass their genetic characteristics on to their children, the human eye has largely ceased to evolve. It is no longer under constant pressure to improve. In the more industrialized nations during the past several centuries there has probably been a decrease in the general level of man's vision. If it were possible, a comparison between the eyesight of today's young people and that of pioneering era youngsters would be interesting.

Civilized man's eyes may not be as efficient or have the acuity of primitive man's, but thanks to his technology and artificial aids to vision, modern man can see over vastly greater distances, study what was once invisibly small, and has extended the useful years of his seeing many years beyond their earlier limits. Civilization may interfere with the normal development of natural processes, but often it also provides a generous measure of replacement.

3 The Magic Eye

Belief in the evil eye is one of man's earliest and most pervasive superstitions. Any demon that might occupy a human body could project his evil spells through the eyes. Witches, as well as the spirits of the dead, have been considered able to work their evil spells through the eyes of the living. Often this belief has been used against anyone who was strange or different.

People of different tribes or nations are frequently the first to be suspected of having the evil eye. Outlanders are the first to be blamed when misfortune strikes — drought or flood, unusual heat or cold, famine or plague. Similarly, individuals who are different from the norm are often held suspect. A redhead among dark-haired people, a person with brown eyes where blue eyes are usual; these are potential possessors of the evil eye. People have used a number of protective devices against the evil eye. A common belief, still prevalent today, is that the color red will help ward off this danger. Red ribbons or flowers on an infant's crib or in a person's hair are held to offer a measure of safety.

Many different peoples at different times and places have held similar beliefs about the evil that can be wrought by the eye, and the means of protecting against it. In his monumental work, *The Golden Bough*, Frazer notes that in the Pelew Islands of the southwest Pacific, in western Asia, and on some of the Aegean islands, boys are dressed as girls to avoid the evil eye. Since boys are considered desirable and girls are not, it follows that boys are more likely to arouse the jealous spite of the demons.

Men when they married were also thought to arouse the hostility of envious demons. To protect them from the evil eye and sow confusion among the powers of darkness, the grooms often dressed like women and the brides like men. This ritual of deception was practiced in ancient Sparta, in relatively recent India, among the islanders of the Celebes, and by the Jews living in Egypt during the Middle Ages.

A number of present-day customs had their origin in ancient superstitions, long since forgotten. The idea of a best man at a wedding has such a beginning. The best man, acting as a decoy for the true husband, was intended to draw off the evil eye cast by spirits jealous of their prerogatives. There may even be some validity to the opinion that the medieval custom of *droit du Seigneur* was originally intended to protect the bridegroom from the anger of the gods.

The magical power of the eye to do evil has been held great, but the eye has also been considered a protective force and a potent element of good.

YOUR SIGHT: FOLKLORE, FACT AND COMMON SENSE

In ancient Egypt, the god Horus was believed to have lost an eye in his struggle against the evil god, Set. Miraculously, Horus regained his vision, and the symbol of his eye became a charm to protect the sight and health of the wearer. This protective symbol passed through many transformations, eventually taking on the appearance of the capital letter R with a line crossing its right leg, ℞ — the sign which precedes our medical prescriptions. Thus, the beneficent magic of the eye protects our health to this very day.

Many seafaring peoples, such as the ancient Phoenicians, painted eyes on the prows of their ships so that they could find their way through the storms and hazards of the seas, and even the present-day Maltese and Portuguese follow this practice.

The eyes, as "windows of the soul," have also been associated with personality and character. Many people, though firmly believing themselves to be utterly without superstition or prejudice, are convinced that they can judge a person by the appearance of his eyes. People who are "shifty-eyed" are considered untrustworthy, while those who can "look you straight in the eye" are held to be reliable. (Obviously, any accomplished and successful liar must therefore be one who *can* look you straight in the eye.) People who look at the world through narrowed or "squinty" eyes are sometimes considered dishonest, treacherous, or cruel. The fact is that squinting has little to do with character, but is generally due to defective vision. People whose eyes do not adjust readily for near or far vision often find that their eyes automatically narrow in an effort to correct for the defect.

Nevertheless, facts are too often less persuasive than fancies, and people are too often judged by the shape of their eyes, their color, their appearance.

The absurdities this can lead to may be estimated by considering some precepts on the subject that were put into print in 1856 by Joseph Turnley. In his book, *The Language of the Eye,* published in London, Turnley wrote:

Blue eyes are more significant of gentleness and yielding than brown or black.

Strength, manhood and thought are associated more with brown than with blue eyes.

A man with small ears must have large, noble eyes or he is full of conceit.

Eyes with long, sharp corners which do not turn downward are sanguine and indicative of genius.

No less absurd are some of the beliefs, prejudices, and superstitions that prevail today in various parts of the world. Among some of the dark-eyed primitive peoples of southeast Asia, blue eyes are considered the mark of demons. In the United States, among some of the primitive people in the backwoods of Arkansas and Oklahoma, women may also be judged by the color of their eyes. Gray-eyed women are considered wise, black-eyed women are mettlesome, green-eyed women need tight control, blue-eyed women are faithful. An old local poem declares: "If a woman's eyes are brown, never let your own fall down."

The idea that the eyes are imbued with special powers apart from mere sight is a pervasive one that has existed from earliest times to the present, and among all races of man.

4 From the Earliest View

Man's superstitions have developed over the millions of years he has been on earth, but his recorded knowledge is probably less than eight thousand years old.

Certainly the people of Sumer, who are said to have developed writing, knew about the eye, investigated it, made records of their findings. From what is known of the medicine and science of Sumer, Lagash, Akkad, and those other cities that first arose on the fertile Mesopotamian plain, however, the earliest observations were heavily tinged with the magical overtones of religion. In time, more objective studies were made, records of which exist in the Egyptian papyri.

FROM THE EARLIEST VIEW

As in most primitive civilizations, the curing of illness and the easing of pain were somehow associated with divinity. There were healing gods. Toth, for example, the first of Egypt's healing gods, was a specialist in what the ancient records say was one of the most common complaints, ophthalmia, a severe inflammation of the eye. Those close to the gods — kings and priests — were endowed with some reflection of godlike powers. Thus, in the early days of civilization, gods, kings, and priests were held to be the healers of man's ills, and so were revered.

In Egypt, even in the earliest dynasties, medicine was relatively far advanced and medical records were meticulously kept. A number of these have survived in the various papyri.

In the Ebers Papyrus, a collection of medical writings copied in 1553 B.C. from a series of earlier works dating to perhaps 3000 B.C., there is a record of a physician named Hwy, known as "the Greatest of the Seers." Hwy, who lived about 4000 B.C., is credited with a remedy for an eye disease, possibly the first existing prescription for such an ailment known to man.

Perhaps half a millennium after Hwy, in 3500 B.C., according to the Ebers Papyrus, diseases of the eye were already a medical specialty in Egypt, with the physician Ypy bearing the title "Consultant of the Palace to Heal the Sight."

Medical specialization was so well established in Egypt that the historian Herodotus commented: "each physician applies himself to only one disease and no more. All parts abound in physicians. There are physicians for the eyes, others for the head, others for the teeth, others for the intestines, others for internal disturbances." There were even specialists, known as "Shepherds of the Rectum," who dealt only with the lower bowel.

The very earliest Egyptian medicine, which was less involved with religion, magic, and superstition than the later medicine of Egypt, was of an unusually high order, and in some respects was not matched until relatively recent times. For this reason it is not surprising that the remedies for eye troubles, listed in the Ebers Papyrus and dating back perhaps five thousand years, might be no less effective than remedies used in Europe a century or so ago. A remedy for eye inflammation is worth repeating, if only for its interest: "To drive away inflammation of the eyes, have ground the stems of the juniper of Byblos, have them steeped in water and apply it to the eyes of the sick person and he will be quickly cured."

Many of the Ebers prescriptions, as well as a number of those in the other medical papyri of Egypt, would be considered effective today. Others that might have been effective cannot be prepared because of problems of translation. A number of the names of plants, herbs, and other substances used by the Egyptians are unknown to us, and consequently cannot be identified.

The Egyptians also made the earliest known artificial eyes, but used them to adorn statues and mummies. Artificial eyes found in mummies might conceivably have served as replacements during life, but no evidence has yet been found to support this conjecture.

The artificial eyes of Egypt were often made of silver, covered over with a white enamel. The iris was represented by a brown ring, with a black dot as the pupil. Occasionally, such eyes have been found with a white pupil, which may have been an effort to show, symbolically, the presence of a cataract.

Cataract, no less a problem today than in primitive times, was treated surgically by the Egyptians in a way not very much different in effect from the treatment of today. The renown of the Egyptians as the first great eye specialists was well deserved; in addition to treating a number of serious eye ailments medically, their surgery was well advanced. The skill of these Nilotic healers was so widely famed, in fact, that Egyptian specialists were sometimes called upon to treat notables in distant lands, as a tablet in the British Museum attests. Cyrus, king of Persia, this record tells us, imported an Egyptian specialist to treat the eyes of his mother.

Realizing that the clouded lens was the culprit that impeded vision, the Egyptians got it out of the way by pushing it aside. This operation was known as couching, and it was performed thousands of years ago. Today, the lens is removed altogether rather than pushed aside, but the same goal is accomplished, permitting light to pass unobscured to the retina.

The couching operation for cataract became widely used by the Greeks and Romans, then by medieval Arab surgeons, who passed along the technique to western Europe. There is even evidence that such an operation was practiced by the Inca and Aztec physicians, as well as by other early peoples who apparently had no known contact with the Egyptians or their surgical heirs.

This appearance of knowledge in separated locales apparently unrelated to each other is one of the surprising characteristics of human history. Herbs containing salycilates — the drug in aspirin — were used by primitive people in the Americas, Africa, the Pacific Islands, Asia, and Europe. Identical beliefs and almost identical rituals concerning hunting, fishing, sowing, and reaping have leaped the barriers of space, time, and race almost since the very first man appeared on earth. So perhaps it should not be surprising that the couching operation may have been developed independently by different people in different places at different times. Wherever or whenever he exists, man remains man, and faced with similar problems he is often likely to find similar answers.

Another early development in medicine that made an impact lasting to this very day is the Code of Hammurabi. Hammurabi, a king of Babylon who ruled about 1900 B.C., drew up a set of laws which, among other things, regulated the practice of medicine. He not only defined the responsibilities of the physician toward the patient, but even established a standard set of fees.

A remarkable aspect of this code is the light it sheds upon the importance of maladies of the eye at that early period of civilization. In Babylonia as in Egypt, the eye and its problems was of major concern. Decreed Hammurabi: "If a physician . . . shall open an abscess with the operating knife and save the eye of the patient, he shall usually be given ten shekels of silver. If it is a slave whose eye is treated, his master shall usually pay two shekels of silver to the physician.

"If a physician . . . shall open an abscess with an operating knife and destroy the eye, his hands shall be cut off."

The Code of Hammurabi, rigorously enforced, may have tended to prevent unnecessary operations; and even to discourage some necessary ones.

Some thirty-five hundred years after Hammurabi, medieval Europe saw the glimmering of scientific medicine as it began its emergence from the Dark Ages. A school was formed in Salerno, on the island of Sicily, under the aegis of the enlightened Emperor Frederick II, King of Sicily and Jerusalem. Frederick, like Hammurabi, set up a code of medical practice, decreed rigid standards for the teaching of medicine, and even required that physicians be licensed to practice.

Much of the medicine taught at Salerno was the scientific medicine developed by the Egyptians and Greeks. This learning had been sent into exile for over a thousand years to make way for the religious healing of the early Christians, but fortunately, the knowledge had been preserved and advanced by the Arabs and Jews.

In 1480, some 240 years after the school of Salerno was established, a medical poem appeared that was said to contain the core of all the practical medical writings up until that time. The poem, *Regimen Sanitatis Salernitanum,* consisted of as many as 3,520 verses, including one devoted to eyesight:

> Now you shall see what harmful is for sight:
> Wine, women, baths, by art to nature wrought,
> Leeks, onions, garlic, mustard-seed, fire and light,
> Smoke, bruises, dust, pepper to powder brought,
> Beans, lentils, strains, wind, tears and sunlight bright,
> And all things sharp our eyesight do molest:
> Yet watching hurts them more than all the rest.

How women, baths, and watching, or using the eyes, "our eyesight do molest" can only be explained as remnants of Dark Ages ignorance. Still, for its time and the darkness it sought to illuminate, the Salernan poem was a remarkable achievement.

But long before Europe was struggling out of the self-imposed "blessed" ignorance of the Dark Ages, the medical school of Hippocrates, which was located on the Aegean island of Cos, had already advanced the idea that the brain was the center of sensation. This in itself was a revolutionary concept at the time: the fifth century B.C. Sight, the Hippocratic physicians believed, resulted from the formation of an image on the pupil of the eye, and this was somehow sensed by the brain.

An equally startling concept, but scientifically accurate nonetheless, was the one advanced by the Arab physician known to the West as Alhazen of Basra, a city in southern Persia. Alhazen, who lived from A.D. 965 to 1039, is justly considered one of the great pioneers in the field of optics. His main work, *On Optics,* showed what was for the time a profound understanding of the functions of the eye. He even experimented with magnifying glasses, and is believed by some medical historians to have made an important contribution to the development of eyeglasses.

Prior to Alhazen, it had been generally believed that the eye saw by sending some mysterious visual ray out *to* the object being viewed. But Alhazen declared that the reverse was true. What the eye actually saw were the visual rays coming *from* the object.

It was not until the Renaissance that Europe, using the knowledge handed down by the Arabs, began once more to explore and expand the realms of knowledge. One of the most unusual figures of that rich period, and one of the least remembered, was Fra Paolo Sarpi of Venice, whose genius reached into mathematics, medicine, astronomy, optics, and even politics. In astronomy, Galileo referred to Fra Paolo, who first used the telescope to map the moon, as "my father and my master." Fabrizio d'Aquapendente, the teacher of William Harvey, called the Venetian friar "medicine's oracle of the century." The Republic of Venice, engaged in a dispute with the Vatican over the separation of church and state, appointed the remarkable Fra Paolo its theological consultant, thus earning him the wrath of the Holy Inquisition. In optics Fra Paolo Sarpi, whom his enemies dubbed "the terrible friar," dissected the eye and discovered the actions and functions of the iris in regulating the amount of light permitted to fall on the lens. He passed his findings along to his friend Fabrizio, who was professor of anatomy at the University of Padua, and who taught them to his students.

At about the same time, in Germany, a major contribution to man's knowledge of sight was being made by the astronomer Johannes Kepler. In 1611, he published a treatise entitled *Dioptrice* in which he declared the retina to be the part of the eye most directly responsible for vision.

In various other writings he included additional important observations. He noted that the lens was an elastic structure that focused the light upon the sensitive retina; he also showed that an abnormally short eye caused farsightedness and an abnormally long eye caused nearsightedness.

The noted French philosopher-scientist René Descartes next took the scientific exploration of the eye a great step forward. The matter of vision came under his investigation in 1637 when he compared the eye to the *camera obscura* — a box with a lens at one end and a screen for the image at the other — and matched the structural similarities between the organ of sight and this early camera. He did additional work clarifying the function of the crystalline lens in focusing light upon the sensitive part of the retina, which he named the *fovea*. The image, or pattern of light impulses, thus formed was transmitted to the brain via the optic nerve. This nerve, he found, seemed to spread out after it entered the eye, and actually formed the major portion of the retina itself.

Many other scientists before and after Descartes studied the existing knowledge and used it as a tool with which additional understanding could be gained. What is known about the eye and vision today is the product of the efforts of numberless men, from the first tentative observations of the near-human creature who crossed the threshold to humanity to the most sophisticated findings of present-day scientists.

This tapestry of understanding is by no means complete. There are many areas still to be filled in — the nature of light itself, for instance; or the specific mechanisms of visual interpretation and recall as they take place in the brain. But scientists today do know much about the structure of the eye and the mechanics of its operation. They also know a good deal about what can go wrong, how to prevent some of these malfunctions and how to correct a number of them.

5 The Seeing Eye

Anyone reading the words on this page is doing far more than simply "seeing." Instead, almost automatically and without conscious awareness, he is performing a series of incredibly complex acts.

Unlike *Euglena viridis,* whose simple eye and nervous system can only detect the difference between varying degrees of light and darkness, man's eyes can determine form, contour, size, color, distance, and fine details. This requires a highly elaborate eye, as well as a sophisticated method of evaluating and interpreting what is seen. The vast number of points of light and dark that make up an image projected upon the retina must be processed by that most compact of all computers, the human brain, so that man can know what it is that he is seeing, evaluate it, and act upon the information appropriately.

When René Descartes compared the eye to the *camera obscura,* the analogy was acceptable but inadequate. The advanced modern camera is a somewhat better comparison. Consider the eye as a self-adjusting, fully automatic, color motion picture camera that instantly develops and projects the image it receives. Like any camera, it requires light, which actually is all that it can "see." In a camera, the light comes in at the front, is focused by the lens, and is directed to the photosensitive film or plate at the back. The eye does precisely this, and much more.

Light coming from an object enters the front of the eye and passes through the pupillary opening to the lens, which focuses it upon the retina at the back of the eye. This light falls upon the retinal screen in a pattern that is equivalent to the pattern of light coming from the object being looked at.

As the light pattern falls upon the retina, it stimulates light-sensitive cells, which react by discharging bursts of electrochemical energy that are in turn carried by the optic nerve to the "seeing" centers of the brain. These bursts of energy are, in effect, a coded message that describes the light pattern on the retina. The brain decodes the message, interprets it, and then tells our consciousness what it is that we are seeing.

The human eye maintains a unique balance between utility and safety, effectively performing its function of seeing and at the same time remaining reasonably protected from hazards. One of the eye's first lines of protection is the socket within which it rests, a bony cavity called the *orbit*. Except for the frontal opening through which the eye sees, and several openings in the back for blood vessels and nerves, the eye is completely enclosed by the orbit.

The surface of the bony orbit is lined by a tough, protective membrane called the *periosteum;* and the six muscles that move the eye are attached at their far ends to a ligament at the back of the orbital cavity. Within this protective cave, the eye is separated from the bone by a thick layer of semiliquid fat. This acts as a shock absorber, cushioning the delicate globe of the eye against damage from blows and the shock of violent movement.

The front of the eye, exposed because of the needs of seeing, has another system of self-defense. First are the eyelids, which can cover the eye to prevent the entry of foreign bodies or damaging light rays, and also provide a certain amount of protection against excessive heat, cold, fluids, and gases. On the inner surface of both eyelids there is a delicate membranous lining called the *conjunctiva*. This membrane completely covers the interior of the lids as well as the exposed cornea at the front of the eyeball. As the lids open and close over the eye, the protective layers of conjunctiva slide over each other, preventing irritation.

Naturally, since the eyelids move over the eyeball with considerable frequency, the conjunctival surfaces need lubrication. This is provided by tears, a fluid continuously secreted in small amounts by the *lacrimal glands* that lie under the bone just above the upper and outer portion of each eye. The tears flow over the surface of the eye, cleaning as well as lubricating it. In addition, tears provide a certain amount of protection against bacteria; they have been found to contain a substance called *lysozyme,* which is known to have antibacterial properties. After the tears have spread over the surface of the eye and inner eyelids, they are drained off through small tubes, called *lacrimal ducts,* at the inner corner of each eye.

People think of tears in terms of sorrow and weeping, but their primary purpose is to protect, rather than to express emotions. Without tears to lubricate and clean the exposed surface of the eyeball, the conjunctiva would dry up, become irritated and inflamed, and the eye itself would be destroyed.

ANATOMY OF THE EYE

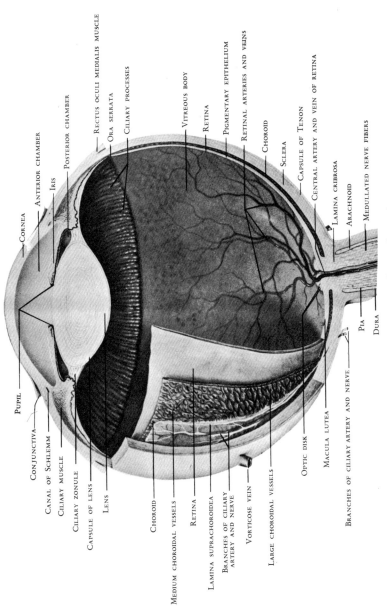

Adapted from original illustration by Paul Peck for Lederle Laboratories

THE LIDS AND LACRIMAL SYSTEM

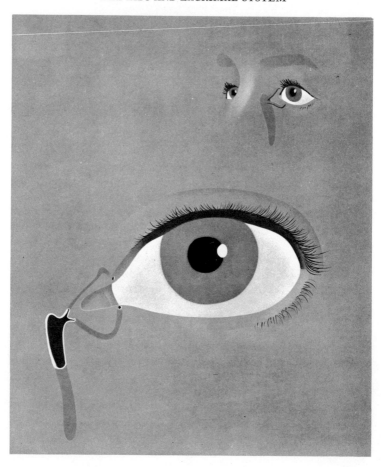

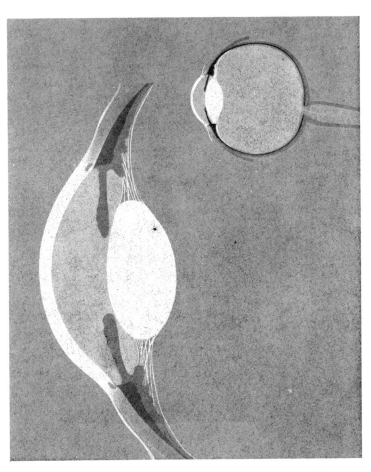

ANTERIOR CHAMBER, LENS AND ANGLE STRUCTURES

THE RETINA

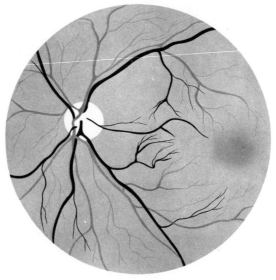

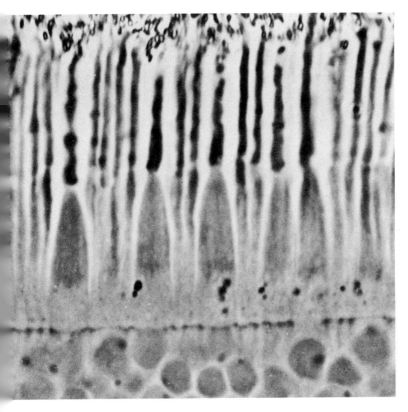

Rods and cones of a human eye as seen under electron microscope by Dr. John E. Dowling, Wilmer Ophthalmological Institute, Johns Hopkins University.

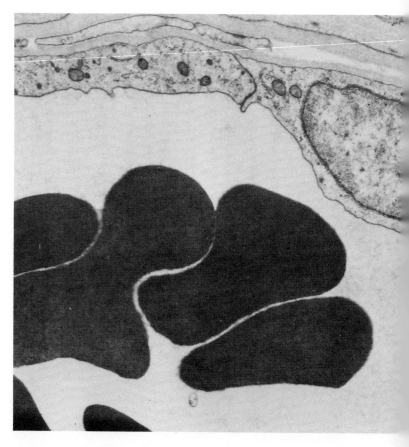

Human blood vessel of the retina as seen under high magnification of electron microscope by Dr. John E. Dowling, Wilmer Ophthalmological Institute, Johns Hopkins University.

THE MUSCLES OF THE EYE

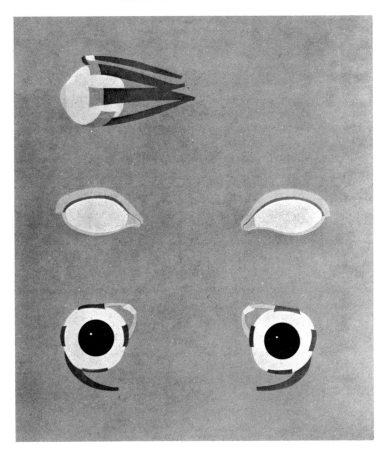

YOUR SIGHT: FOLKLORE, FACT AND COMMON SENSE

Nearly spherical in shape and about 0.94 of an inch in diameter, the eye is truly a miracle of natural miniaturization, as if a sophisticated motion picture camera and projector were built into a sphere somewhat smaller than a golf ball. The eye is constructed in several layers, each one performing a very special function. The layers at the front are somewhat different from those at the back, since front and back have different tasks.

The job of the outer layer of the eye is largely protective. The tough, transparent membrane at the front of the eye is called the *cornea*, and its smooth, regular curve is very important to the effective function of the eye's optical system. Differences and irregularities in the curve of the cornea will distort the light that enters the eye, and can produce astigmatism or even more serious defects in vision. The remainder of the protective outer layer, called the *sclera*, extends from the cornea to the back of the eyeball. This is the "white" of the eye, a fibrous tissue that is opaque and flexible.

The layer beneath the cornea-sclera is called the *uvea*, and it, too, is composed of a front and rear portion. The front part consists of the colored portion of the eye, the *iris*, and the *ciliary body*, a ring of muscles and blood vessels located at the base of the iris. Both the iris and ciliary body perform the highly important task of regulating the amount of light that enters the eye.

Behind this forward portion of the uvea, ranging along the sides and back of the eye, is the rest of the uveal layer, known as the *choroid*. The choroid carries a great number of blood vessels that bring oxygen and nutrients into the eye and carry off wastes.

Finally, lying like a cup along the sides and rear of the eye, is the innermost layer, the *retina*.

While the two outer layers of the eye protect and nourish the organ of sight, the optical system that collects and focuses the light we see by extends in a line from the front of the eye to the back. At the very front, as we noted, is the clear window of the cornea, through which light enters the eye. Behind the cornea, separated by a space, is the colored iris, with its central opening, the pupil. Then there is another space, beyond which lies the *crystalline lens* that focuses the light upon the retina at the rear of the eye.

Filling the spaces between cornea and iris and iris and lens is a fluid called the *aqueous humor*. This fluid is normally maintained at a constant pressure, which among other things helps the cornea preserve its proper curvature. If for some reason the pressure of the aqueous humor increases, the serious disease known as *glaucoma* may result.

The major portion of the eye's interior, the space between the lens and the retina, is filled with a transparent jellylike substance called the *vitreous humor*. By maintaining outward pressure, the vitreous acts to keep the various layers of the eye in their proper position and in contact with each other.

So much for the general structure of the eye. As a piece of rational engineering it seems simple and straightforward, but when we consider each of the separate elements of the eye, what they do and how they do it, the complexities are almost beyond description.

Iris and Pupil

Everyone needs light to see, but too much light can be damaging to the eye. This is especially true of ultraviolet light, a component of sunlight, which can cause serious injury to the lens and retina. Here, too, there is a close similarity to the camera. If too much light enters, the film is overexposed and the picture "burns out"; but if insufficient light enters, the film will be underexposed and the picture will be very faint, if it shows at all.

The automatic camera is guarded against over- and underexposure by proper adjustment of the lens opening, which is stopped down in bright light and opened wide in dim. In the human eye, the light-regulating apparatus works very much the same way. The iris opens and closes, depending upon the amount of available light. As it opens, the pupil — the actual opening through which light passes to the lens — becomes larger. As the iris closes, the pupil becomes smaller.

The eye's sensitive light-regulating system resembles a built-in exposure meter in a camera. As light enters the eye, its intensity is immediately measured by nerves in the retina, which sends a feedback signal to the delicate ciliary muscles that control the iris. These muscles then relax or contract, increasing or reducing the size of the pupil to admit the light required.

Iris and pupil are in a constant state of adjustment and readjustment. However wide open the pupil may be, though, little if anything can be seen when there is too little light to start with; and if we stare into such a powerful light source as the sun, our eyes will be damaged no matter how tiny the pupils become. Sunlight focused through a glass lens can scorch wood or burn a hole in paper. The same sunlight, focused through the lens of the eye, can burn the retina and injure the lens as well.

The Lens

The lens, properly called the crystalline lens, is a transparent, elastic, biconvex structure built up of clear protein cells, densely packed together in a highly orderly fashion. Its focusing ability depends upon a membranous capsule that encloses it. This capsule is kept at varying degrees of tension by a ring of muscles that are part of the ciliary body, and their tension in turn is controlled by feedback mechanisms resembling those that open and close the iris. As we look at an object, the nervous system sends signals back from the retina to the muscle fibers, changing the tensions of the lens membrane. This adjusts the curvature to bring the object into the sharpest possible focus. Thus, the eye's lens changes focus by changing its shape. Curving sharply on both sides, the not quite spherical lens of the eye flattens its curve to bring distant objects into focus, or increases its curve to view close objects. This process of automatic focusing is known as *accommodation*.

As we age, the lens becomes more densely packed with cells and begins to lose flexibility. In addition, age weakens the muscles that help the lens change its shape. Most people past the age of forty find they need corrective glasses to compensate for the declining ability of the lens to focus. When the lens becomes packed with an abnormal density of cells, or the cells lose their transparency, a cataract may develop.

The Retina

All the other parts of the eye's optical system — the cornea, the iris, the lens — exist to bring light to the sensitive surface of the retina, the screen upon which the lens focuses the light we see. As already noted, the retina was originally a part of the brain itself, a collapsed bubble that has taken the shape of a cup at the end of the optic nerve. At the surface of the retina, facing the lens, there are a vast number of pigmented nerve cells that are sensitive to light. These are called *rods* and *cones,* and although they look alike when seen through an electron microscope, they seem to serve different purposes, apparently because of chemical differences in the pigments they contain. Rods are more sensitive to light than cones, and play an important role in helping people see in dim light. Cones are important in color vision. All of these pigmented cells, the rods and the cones, are linked by a complicated network of nerve cells and fibers to the optic nerve, which transmits the light patterns received by the retina to the visual centers of the brain.

Let us explore the way in which light, falling upon a rod or cone in the retina, is coverted into a signal that can be carried along the nerve network to the brain.

The light-sensitive pigment in the rods and cones is chemically linked to a molecule of protein. This combination of carotenoid pigment and protein holds together when there is no light falling upon it; but when light is present, the combination becomes unstable and separates, releasing a minute amount of energy as it breaks apart. This released energy takes the form of an electrochemical impulse — the signal carried along the chain of nerves to the brain.

The greatest concentration of light-sensitive cells, capable of sending the most detailed visual information to the brain, is in the *macula lutea,* a small yellow-orange area of the retina directly opposite the pupil. Here visual acuity is at its greatest, being particularly sharp in the *fovea centralis,* a tiny depression in the macula.

The Moving Eyeball

The camera has one distinct advantage over the eye; the image it focuses upon a film or photographic plate is equally clear throughout most of the picture. The image focused by the eye's lens upon the retina is sharply defined only in the small section within the macula lutea. The rest of the image loses detail.

Unlike the camera, the human eye has to scan a page or a face or a scene in order to see the details clearly. In reading, for example, the word upon which the eyes are fixed is clear in sharp detail, and so perhaps are a few more surrounding it. The others will not be clearly visible until the eyes are moved so that the image of each word falls upon the macula. Unless the eyes kept moving (as they do almost constantly, without our realizing it) we would actually see very little clearly.

To scan properly, the eye must be freely movable within its

socket. Each eye has six muscles attached to it, arranged in a balanced combination, making possible vertical, horizontal, and oblique movements that give the eye mobility in every necessary direction. As a result, the eyes are able to scan a scene, bringing each detail into clear view on the macula lutea and its point of sharpest vision, the fovea centralis.

Another characteristic that in some ways reduces the efficiency of the eyes is the tendency of the retina to retain each image for about a tenth of a second. While images are transmitted continuously from the retina to the cerebral cortex, a portion of the brain that deals with incoming information, there is a constant overlap. For this reason human eyes are unable to separate clearly a series of rapidly changing images, or to see the precise details of a swiftly moving object, such as the individual spokes of a turning bicycle wheel. It is this "persistence of vision" that enables us to enjoy motion pictures. Without it, the frames would not overlap and run together to create the illusion of continuous motion; each would be seen as a distinct and disconnected picture.

Three-Dimensional Sight

Our two eyes, with their lenses approximately three inches apart, actually see two images of each object. The left eye sees slightly more of the left side, the right eye of the right, and the brain ordinarily superimposes the two images over one another to create what appears to be a single three-dimensional view of what we are looking at. This process is known as *fusion,* and helps provide us with depth perception in addition to stereoscopic vision.

We are visually aware of a wide area above, below, and to the sides of the primary object seen in sharp focus. The boundary of all that we see, while our eyes are fixed straight ahead, is known as the *limit of peripheral vision,* and everything seen within that boundary is the *field of vision.*

To test your field of vision, extend your arms straight out in front of your eyes, fists clenched and thumbs pointed up. Look straight ahead at the thumbs, so they are in sharp focus, and move your arms slowly outward as far as you can and still see both thumbs simultaneously. Your field of vision lies between the two thumbs when they are both still visible.

Most people have a field of vision equal to a little more than half a circle, somewhat better than 180 degrees. Outside of this field of vision is what is called a *blind zone.* Birds, whose eyes are placed on the sides rather than the front of the head, have no blind zone, and can see what is behind them as well as what is in front.

The field of vision not only differs somewhat from person to person, but can also vary in the same person at different times. Tests by Yale University researchers have shown that alcohol, for instance, can decrease peripheral vision. A single drink can reduce a driver's field of vision sufficiently to prevent his seeing an object coming from the side until too late to avert an accident. Other chemical substances, illness, and cigarette smoke also reduce the field of vision, as does the aging process. Such reductions of the field of vision are temporary, except when caused by certain illnesses or aging.

Within the field of vision of each eye there is one small area that will show no image, known as the *blind spot.* An image cast upon the part of the retina occupied by the beginning of the optic nerve cannot be seen, because this nerve, which transmits visual images to the brain, cannot produce them. It consists of the nerve fibers that are gathered from the rest of the retina, and has no light-sensitive rods and cones.

The blind spot can be demonstrated by a simple experiment.

Make two dots about two and a half inches apart on a sheet of white paper. Close the left eye and look steadily at the left dot, holding the paper about ten inches in front of the right eye. Then move the paper slowly toward the eye. At some point, as you move the paper, the right dot will disappear, as its image falls on the optic nerve. As you move the paper still closer the dot will reappear, because its image has moved off the optic nerve to a light-sensitive portion of the retina.

Seeing in Color

Color depends upon the frequency or wavelength of light coming from an object. The longest wavelength in the visible spectrum is that of red, followed in decreasing order by orange, yellow, green, blue, indigo, and violet. That much has been established by the physicists and can be shown experimentally. Much less clear is the manner in which color is seen. At present there are a number of theories which seem to have one underlying premise. This is the concept that there are three types of color-sensitive cones in the human retina, one sensitive to red, another to green, and the third to blue-violet. These cones are stimulated by light of the appropriate frequency.

When light enters the eyes and stimulates all three types of cones equally, we see white. If only one type of cone is stimulated, the color to which this cone is sensitive is seen. Since there are no cones sensitive to orange and yellow, these colors are seen when light stimulates the cones adjoining them on both sides of the color spectrum — the red-sensitive cones on one side and the green-sensitive on the other.

Therefore, when red- and green-sensitive cones are stimulated to an appropriately balanced degree, yellow is seen. Orange is seen if there is greater stimulation of the red-sensitive cones, and yellow-green, or chartreuse, is seen if there is greater stimulation of the green-sensitive cones.

The manner in which the color frequencies received by the retina are mixed and interpreted by the brain is considerably different from the way in which an artist blends pigments, and the two processes cannot be usefully compared.

Color vision, of course, is far from equal in everyone, and can suffer some derangements. A reversible form of color blindness can be produced in some individuals by inhaled tobacco smoke. At the University of Washington in Seattle recently, Dr. P. J. Fialkow and his associates conducted a series of experiments which showed that both alcohol and certain types of liver disease, particularly cirrhosis, also produce a form of red-green color blindness. In most cases, vision returns to normal once the system rids itself of the alcohol or the liver disease.

Between the two events of looking and seeing, a vast number of interrelated actions must take place, the failure of any of which might distort, damage, or block our ability to see. We can summarize the process. Light from an object enters the eye at the cornea, triggering a feedback signal from the retina that causes the iris to open or close, depending upon the intensity of the light coming from the object. Passing through the adjusted pupillary opening, the light next falls upon the lens which, in response to another set of impulses and feedback signals, corrects its curvature to bring the object into correct focus. The light then passes from the lens through the transparent vitreous and casts its focused pattern upon the light- and color-sensitive cells of the retina. Because of the light now falling upon them, the pigments in these rod and cone cells separate from their binding proteins, and the consequent release of energy sets up a pattern of neural signals equivalent to the object that is being observed. These signals are carried by nerve fibers in the retina to the optic nerve, then along the optic nerve to the cortex of the brain, where the image of the object is finally perceived.

That, fundamentally, is how we see.

Color Blindness

Although color blindness is a generally used term, widely accepted in describing a defect in color vision, it is basically inaccurate; the color-blind person does see the object in question, but he may not be able to perceive its correct hue.

The most common such defect results in an inability to perceive red or green, sometimes both. Much more rare is the inability to distinguish blue. The reasons for this defect are not clear, although it is widely believed that hereditary factors are involved, with the affected retinas lacking some of the elements necessary to generate an appropriate response to color sensitization. Occasionally, green blindness is known to be a temporary result of smoking. Men are much more frequently affected than women.

For the most part, green-blind persons see a grayish hue instead of green. Red-blind people cannot see a red square on a black field, and often confuse red with green or brown. They will not see the red in colors that contain a red component, such as orange or purple. Instead, purple will appear blue, and orange will be seen as yellow. Similarly, green-blind persons will see turquoise as pure blue, and chartreuse as yellow.

Genetic studies now under way may make it possible to learn the precise defect responsible for this flaw in color vision. Most likely, it is suspected, it is due to a missing or defective enzyme. If this is correct, it is not outside the range of possibility that the defect could be corrected by the developing techniques of genetic manipulation.

6 Recognition

We look at a face and we "see" it; its nose, eyes, forehead, mouth, and chin. We are aware of a pictorial representation of the person. To us, this has recognizable reality. Yet all that our eyes have actually received from this face is its reflected light. Had there been no light to reflect, we would have seen no face.

On the retina, the light from the face is focused to produce patterns of electrochemical discharges that are sent to the brain in the form of neural signals. At no point in this process has the lens, the retina, or the brain received a "picture." Instead, the face we are "seeing" consists of a complex arrangement of coded signals that the brain must interpret, recognize, and then translate into information that is projected into our consciousness in the form of a picture. What we really are "seeing" is the characteristic and specific perceptual response we have to a particular pattern of visual impulses.

Anyone who has ever been struck on or near the eye and "seen stars" will find it easier to understand that people actually "see" their own responses to optic stimuli, not the objects causing the stimuli.

As we have already noted, the light-sensitive cells of the retina discharge an electrochemical impulse when light falls upon them. This impulse is transmitted to the appropriate part of the brain by the optic nerve and produces the "seen" mental image.

The violent stimulus of a blow also causes the light-sensitive cells of the retina to discharge their neural impulses. Since these impulses are conducted by the optic nerve to the portion of the brain dealing with vision, they are interpreted as a visual experience and flashes of light are "seen."

There are other ways of producing false visual experiences or hallucinations, and these provide some insights into how the brain and nervous system work.

In 1958, Dr. Wilder Penfield of McGill University in Montreal performed what has become a classic experiment. He sent mild impulses of electricity into the brains of a number of individuals suffering from epilepsy. These harmless electric charges were directed into a specific portion of the cerebral cortex where memories are stored. Stimulated by the current, the brain cells released their memories into the consciousness, not as memories of past events but as new experiences being lived at the moment. The people receiving the charges not only heard the sounds of the past experiences as though they were taking place in the present, but even saw the sights of those past events as though their eyes were viewing them at that moment.

Certainly it would seem from this and other information that

YOUR SIGHT: FOLKLORE, FACT AND COMMON SENSE

the eye does not "see." Its task is to collect light from specific objects and translate them into patterns of nerve signals, which the brain then interprets and pictures for our consciousness. It is the brain, not the eye, that does the visualizing and produces the image of what we see.

The brain that accomplishes this task is a compact biological computer which can not only process data but can program and direct itself, learning as it functions. It has inputs, outputs, storage areas where memories are kept and even stored in duplicate. It also possesses delicate switching mechanisms and relays, as well as an incredibly complex web of connecting circuits and networks.

The giant computer may have several million electronic elements in the form of tubes, transistors, diodes, and so on — the human brain has an estimated *one thousand billion* neural elements. Its switching time, speeding impulses from one group of elements to another, is estimated in ten-thousandths of a second.

The brain is involved in virtually every aspect of our actions, from managing fundamental reflexes and controlling the essential processes of life — breathing, blood circulation, digestion, metabolism, growth — to thinking, feeling, remembering, processing the information provided by our senses, and all of the so-called higher functions and creative processes.

To function efficiently, the brain keeps in constant touch with its environment, internal as well as external. It is continuously receiving data about the oxygen and nutriment needs of each organ and tissue of the body, and through the senses of smell, touch, taste, hearing, and sight, the portion of the brain known as the *cortex* receives information about conditions in the external environment. Without this constant flow of information to be processed, interpreted, and acted upon by the brain and central nervous system man would be unable to survive, and would probably never even have evolved.

This small but indispensable computer, fitting neatly inside the skull, is so complex that during an average second of its activity it performs approximately five trillion operations, each one of which is associated with the discharge of an electrochemical impulse. Just as it visualizes optical data, it also "hears," "smells," "tastes," and "feels."

Information sent to the cortex from the eyes is undoubtedly more complicated than that sent from other organs of sense. There are approximately one million nerve fibers in the retina, each one sending bits of data which the brain must interpret, evaluate, make available for recall, and possibly act upon.

It would be physically impossible for the brain to process fully each bit of data provided by the eyes. The cortex, which is concerned with relating us to external environment, has, over the eons of evolution, developed a relatively efficient way of handling this problem: Instead of dealing with each piece of data as a separate entity it treats them as parts of patterns and groups of data bits. The patterns of visual impulses that are discharged by the retina are directed by the optic nerve to the *primary visual receptive cortex,* in the lower portion of the back of the cerebral cortex. These patterns, combined into groups, are then switched to *visual association areas,* located somewhat above the receptive cortex.

In the course of processing, the brain notes the pattern of impulses, codes it, and sends the coded signal to the memory cells. If any identical or similar coded patterns exist, they are released along with associated data — whether danger or pleasure were involved, what sort of reaction was most effective — and the brain uses this and other information to achieve identification of what has been seen. Then the visual image of what the brain tells us we have seen is released to our consciousness, and we react to it. If the visual experience is a new one, with no data in the memory banks, then the brain will make assumptions, probably based on a synthesis of the most closely related associations. These assumptions are modified or expanded as new information and further experience either contradict or confirm them.

Thus, we recognize a face as a face, a bird as a bird, even though the particular one we are looking at is new to us. But if we see something entirely unlike anything we have ever seen, we still can recognize general characteristics — shape, color, size — because such information, covering a vast range of possible experience, is already in our memory cells. Such general information is stored in our memories and, with more data and experience, we can make more precise conclusions about the nature of what we see. This process, infrequent in adults, is basic to the learning of infants, with virtually empty memory banks, to whom each experience is new. When an infant sees an object he reaches out to grasp it, smell it, taste it, listen to its sounds. Gradually all of this information is integrated into a single entity, and the identifying data is stored and cross-indexed in the memory banks. With the development and refinement of the infant's perceptions, he learns to recognize the object with only one set of sensory signals — either by sight, sound, smell, taste, or touch. He will know his mother, for instance, from the sight of her face, the sound of her voice, or one of the other patterns of information.

Since we cannot possibly process and integrate all of the data we receive, we tend to form generalizations about what we see. From these generalizations, our brain selects what appears to be the most appropriate of a series of alternatives. This singled-out alternative then becomes the "seen" object. Should our cortex select the wrong alternative, as occasionally happens, then our eyes are said to have "deceived" us.

During the course of interpreting and identifying what we see, the brain also processes data relating to size and distance. Obviously, a tree fifty feet away seems twice as tall as a tree of equal size one hundred feet away, because the retinal image cast by the nearer tree is twice as big as that cast by the other. Nonetheless, the brain can judge the difference in distance and take into account the apparent difference in size.

Precisely how this is done is not easily explained. Depth perception plays a role, as do past experiences which help us estimate the size-distance relationships of already known objects. More important, perhaps, is the feedback mechanism that adjusts the focus of the lens to the distance of the object being viewed. This process apparently also provides the brain with information regarding relative distances.

The brain also orients the upside-down image pattern cast upon the retina, so that it appears right side up. Furthermore, it coordinates the separate images from each eye, superimposing and adjusting them for minor variations of size and alignment in order to produce the impression of a single image.

The noted University of Moscow psychologist, A. R. Luria, suggests that the process of recognition begins with the identification of one particular sign of an object. From this sign a "perceptual hypothesis" is created, then elaborated or rejected as new signs are selected from a series of alternatives. As the process of recognition draws to completion, the subsidiary, unimportant signs are suppressed and the important signs brought to the foreground of consciousness, where they are integrated into the "recognized" image.

This theory, which suggests that we begin making assumptions about what we are seeing long before we have all the visual data, helps explain how some of the astronauts have been able to see ships' wakes, roads, and even houses that were literally too far away to be seen. Furthermore, it helps us understand how we can recognize a very close friend from a considerably greater distance than a mere acquaintance. Obviously we recognize the friend first because we need fewer visual clues to make an assumption about his identity. The acquaintance, being less familiar, requires more clues for recognition.

Optical Illusions

The part of the brain that interprets what we see is by no means infallable. Certain errors in judging size, shape, color, location, and distance are made by everyone. We know them as *optical illusions*. Vertical lines give the illusion of height, horizontal lines the illusion of width or length. Interior decorators use these optical illusions to make a low room appear taller, a short room longer, or a narrow room wider.

Interesting optical illusions are created by different colors. Each color of the spectrum has a different wavelength, red having the longest and violet the shortest. The long wavelength of red has to be refracted or bent more sharply than the succeedingly shorter wavelengths of orange, yellow, green, blue, indigo, and violet. Therefore, when we look at something red, the lens takes the same shape that it would if we were looking at something close, while a blue or violet object gives the lens the same shape it would take for a distant object. Since the brain judges distance by the shape that the lens must take to bring an object into focus, colors can be deceptive.

Artists use this phenomenon to give the impression of depth to their paintings. A splash of red or orange ("hot" or advancing colors) on a canvas makes that part of the painting seem close, and green and blue ("cool" or receding colors) seem to go off into the distance. Properly used, even without the lines that suggest perspective, colors can create the illusion of three dimensions on a two-dimensional canvas.

To demonstrate this phenomenon, draw a vertical line about half an inch wide and six inches long with a red crayon on a sheet of white paper. On either side of it draw similar orange lines, then

RECOGNITION

yellow lines outside of the orange lines, then green, then blue. If you stand away and look at the result, the red will appear closest, with the other colors seeming to recede.

Fortunately, our eyes do not deceive us often, and when they do the consequences are rarely serious. Instead, the eye-brain complex that really does our seeing correctly recognizes most objects whose light falls upon our eyes. It will tell us how large an object is, how far away, and whether it is approaching or receding. All told, it will provide approximately nine-tenths of all the information we receive from the world around us.

2

THE PROBLEMS OF SIGHT

What the Problems Are 7

The old-fashioned box camera rarely broke down; but it could not be focused sharply, it always needed bright light, and it could only do a fraction of the things that a modern camera can do. The modern camera, with its coupled range finder, built-in light meter, and self-adjusting shutter speed and lens opening, is far more vulnerable, because it has more that can break down. So it is with our eyes. Vulnerability is part of the price we pay for increased complexity and efficiency. With all the things that can go wrong with our eyes, the amazing thing is that so few actually do.

Our eyes, like us, are mortal, and as we age, so do they. Like the rest of the body, the eyes lose efficiency as they grow older.

Fortunately, the sciences of optics and ophthalmology make it possible to compensate for or correct the so-called "degenerative" changes so that, with corrective lenses, we need suffer no significant loss of vision.

Many people think that if they have 20/20 vision their eyes are about as good as they can be. This is not true. All that is meant by 20/20 vision is that at twenty feet we can see what we should be able to see at that distance. Vision rated at 20/30 means that one sees at twenty feet objects that should be clear at thirty. This system of measuring vision was developed in 1863 to be used in conjunction with the standard Snellen eye chart. It does not tell us whether our eyesight is normal; it only measures what we are able to see at twenty feet.

Some people with natural 20/20 vision could not read this page without corrective eyeglasses, and some who need glasses to achieve 20/20 vision could read this page without them. Having 20/20 vision is fine as far as it goes, but it is not enough. For normal vision, one should be able to see clearly and without strain from less than a foot away to infinity.

Care of the eyes and correction of defects in vision rests with a highly trained and skilled group of specialists. First of these is the *ophthalmologist* or *oculist*, who is a medical doctor and surgeon specially qualified to diagnose and treat diseases and defects of the eye. He is also trained to measure changes of vision, whether one is nearsighted or farsighted, and to prescribe corrective lenses.

The *optometrist* is trained and licensed to examine and measure the eyes for defects in vision, to prescribe corrective lenses, and to grind and fit them. While he does not treat diseases of the eye, he is often the first to detect them.

The third specialist is the *optician,* who is trained to grind the lenses prescribed by an ophthalmologist or optometrist, fit them properly, and provide suitable frames for eyeglasses. He does

WHAT THE PROBLEMS ARE

not examine the eyes for visual defects or disease, nor does he treat them.

The division of the problems of sight into two main groups, the ordinary and the extraordinary, is for the author's convenience rather than any scientifically precise distinction. "Ordinary" problems include the effects of the aging process, plus problems and defects that arise mainly from abnormalities in structure — eyeballs that are too large or too small, irregularities of the cornea or lens, defects of the orbital muscles that result in misalignment of the eyes, and so on. These have been called ordinary because they are endogenous and, to a greater or lesser degree, affect all of us. For the most part, too, they are genetically determined, but this distinction is not confined to the ordinary problems.

The "extraordinary" problems, on the other hand, are more likely to be caused by factors outside of ourselves, such as bacterial and viral infections, diseases that affect the eyes, and injuries of one sort or another. This category also includes disturbances that are by-products of various allergic conditions and such ailments as diabetes, hypertension, and gout.

For the most part, these "extraordinary" problems are not genetically influenced to the same degree as the ordinary problems, although heredity certainly plays an indirect role in some, such as diabetes, where the eye involvement is a secondary effect of the disease.

"Ordinary" Problems

Because of the structure of our lenses, two defects are built into all human eyes — *spherical aberration* and *chromatic aberration*. Both defects arise from the fact that the lenses do not bend all light equally. *Spherical aberration,* or *refractive error,* is the slight blurring of the image caused by the fact that not all rays of light come into focus at the same point. Similarly, the different wavelengths of white light are refracted unequally, occasionally causing halos of color, like the bluish haze we see around distant objects. This defect is called *chromatic aberration*.

A third natural defect, *presbyopia* — the inability to focus the eyes clearly on close objects — is an inevitable result of aging. The blind spot on the retina, where the optic nerve begins, could also be called a natural defect, but it does not cause any difficulty because the brain fills this particular gap in our vision with what it assumes we would be seeing there.

Another group of common eye defects arises from variations in the shape of the eyeball, generally hereditary. The normal eyeball is about 1/25 of an inch longer from front to back than it is from side to side or top to bottom. Such a well-proportioned eyeball is called *emmetropic*. Very few eyeballs have perfectly normal dimensions, but the differences are usually so slight that there is no perceptible effect upon vision. The brain makes whatever small adjustments are necessary.

Eyeballs that are significantly longer than they should be cause nearsightedness, or *myopia,* and abnormally short eyeballs cause *hyperopia,* or farsightedness. A third defect belonging to this group, the most common abnormality of all, is *astigmatism,* caused by irregularities in the cornea or the lens or both, resulting in a distorted image cast upon the retina. All of these conditions can be corrected by the use of appropriate eyeglasses or contact lenses.

Less frequent than the defects already mentioned, but by no means rare, is *strabismus,* which involves an imbalance of the six muscles controlling the movements of each eye. (A form of strabismus is also caused by paralysis of one or more of the eye muscles.) The imbalance pulls the eyes out of alignment, causing crossed eyes (*esotropia*), divergent or outward-turning eyes (*exotropia*), or an upward or downward misalignment (*hypertropia* or *hypotropia*).

Strabismus can also create an inability to combine the pictures seen through each eye into a single image. A person so afflicted may see two images, perhaps of two different sizes, and so on. Such disturbances, fortunately rare, may also be the fault of imperfect nerve transmission of the retinal images to the brain, or may even result from errors of interpretation in the cerebral cortex.

When we fail to see things clearly, we may unconsciously tighten or relax the muscles that control the shape of the lens. This is called an *accommodative squint,* since we are attempting to accommodate our vision to the distance of the object.

Finally, there is the condition called *amblyopia,* a dimness or impairment of vision that cannot be attributed to any detectable organic defect, either in the eye itself or in the optic nerve. Some forms of amblyopia are linked to intense emotional disturbances, such as hysteria; to alcoholism; to the toxic effects of arsenic, quinine, and other drugs; to excessive smoking; and even to fatigue.

"Extraordinary" Problems

Glaucoma and cataracts are generally considered the most serious of the "extraordinary" problems. Although it can be controlled, glaucoma is one of the major causes of blindness in the United States, and probably in most of the rest of the world. Yet, with proper care, much of its damage is preventable.

Cataracts also cause blindness in the affected eye. While not preventable, this condition can be corrected to a considerable degree by the removal of the involved lens and the substitution of a contact or other corrective lens.

Besides these two very serious problems there are a number of others that can result in loss or impairment of sight. Various portions of the eye are subject to illness or damage. Some conditions like detached retina, in which the retina comes loose from the choroid against which it normally rests, can be repaired if detected in time. Others, like the retinal damage — retinopathy — that is often seen in diabetes or in high blood pressure, may be extremely difficult to correct. But even in these areas, where the prospect was exceedingly gloomy until recent years, new developments offer considerable hope for improvement.

The eyes are also subject to a series of infections and inflammations, including conjunctivitis, retinitis, uveitis, and papillitis or inflammation of the optic nerve. Various tumors, growths, disturbances of circulation, poisons, and injuries may also threaten our sight, along with hazards from sunlight, ultraviolet, and other radiation, heat, and chemical irritants.

Beyond all these there are a number of degenerative changes, as well as injuries to the brain and other parts of our bodies that can exercise a damaging effect upon our vision. Certain forms of liver disease have been found to produce temporary color blindness; and kidney disease, by interfering with the normal process that purifies the blood, can result in serious eye problems. The blood, after all, provides the eyes as well as the rest of the body with the nutrients and chemicals they need to work properly. If the body's wastes and other toxic materials are not adequately eliminated from the blood, but are instead carried to the eyes, our eyesight is likely to suffer.

Recently, Research to Prevent Blindness, Inc., reported the results of a survey into the causes of blindness in the United States:

Eight out of ten cases of blindness, it was found, result from diseases whose causes are not yet known to science.

Glaucoma, cataract, detached retina, and similar eye diseases of unknown cause are responsible for 38 percent of blindness.

General diseases such as diabetes, hypertension, and other circulatory ills are involved in 16 percent of blindness.

WHAT THE PROBLEMS ARE

In 14 percent of all cases of blindness, the cause was either unknown or unspecified.

Infectious disease was involved in 10 percent of the nation's blindness.

In 9 percent, the cause was unknown but believed to be prenatal in origin.

Injuries were held responsible in 5 percent; hereditary causes in 4 percent, and poisoning in 3 percent.

In only one case of blindness in every hundred was a neoplastic, or cancerous, growth held responsible.

Considering the complexity of our eyes and measuring this against the countless hazards to which they are exposed each day, it is amazing how little actually does go wrong. With a modicum of good sense, care, caution and proper medical attention, most of the dangers can be kept under adequate control.

The chapters that follow will explore the problems of the eye, both "ordinary" and "extraordinary," in detail.

8 Myopia, Hyperopia and Astigmatism

In classic myopia or nearsightedness, objects that are relatively close, from about nine inches to several feet away, are seen clearly, while more distant objects are blurred, sometimes beyond recognition. Extremely myopic people, unless they wear corrective lenses, have to bring objects very close to their eyes in order to see them clearly.

The defect responsible for myopia is an eyeball that is longer than normal. The lens is perfectly normal, refracting the light from objects just as it would for an ordinary eye. However, be-

MYOPIA, HYPEROPIA AND ASTIGMATISM

cause of the eye's extra length, the retina is not where it should be, but further back. As a result, the image is focused in front of the retina instead of on it. The light rays then cross and start to diverge by the time they reach the retina, causing a blurred image.

The further an object is from us, the more nearly parallel are the light rays reaching us from it, while light rays from a close object converge toward us sharply. That is why, for instance, we can see a medium-sized tree one hundred feet away in its entirety, top to bottom, but from only ten feet away, we can no longer take it in at a single glance. This helps explain why distant objects seem blurred to the nearsighted eye. The crystalline lens bends parallel rays more sharply than converging rays. Consequently, the distant object attains its clearest point of focus before its light reaches the retina. Close objects, whose light is not as sharply refracted, are focused directly upon the retina and are clearly seen.

Like the majority of visual defects, nearsightedness is easily overcome with corrective lenses. Concave lenses are used to separate the light rays just before they enter the eye. These separated rays, less sharply refracted than ordinarily, then come to focus upon the retina rather than in front of it.

In hyperopia or farsightedness, the situation is exactly the reverse: the eyeball is too short, and consequently the retina is too far forward. Light from distant objects, which in myopia would come to focus in front of the retina, now reaches the retina in sharp focus — light from near objects comes to focus *behind* the retina. As a result, close objects are blurred and distant objects are clear.

Convex lenses are used to correct hyperopia. These lenses help refract the light from close objects more sharply, so that they can come into focus directly upon the retina. Hyperopic people who do not wear corrective glasses often find themselves holding objects at arm's length in order to be able to see them clearly.

65

Not all light rays are focused to sharp points upon the retina; some form short lines instead. This condition is called *astigmatism*, from a Greek word meaning "without a point," and is common to all of us in one degree or another. Most astigmatism, about 85 percent, is so mild that the brain has little difficulty compensating for it. Of the remaining 15 percent, requiring corrective eyeglasses, all but a small fraction is moderate. Very little, indeed, is severe.

No lens is absolutely perfect, nor is any cornea. That is why all of us have some degree of astigmatism. The curve of a lens or cornea is never precisely accurate throughout; tiny flaws, raised areas, depressions, and other defects, mostly minor ones, distort our vision to some degree. Light passing through one of these flawed areas of cornea or lens will not be bent to the same degree as light passing through a different part, and consequently the rays of light will not meet to form a sharp point upon the retina as they should. Instead they may adjoin or be slightly separated, forming a short line rather than a point.

If our eyes were perfect, stars would appear as sharp pinpoints of light; but since no eye is absolutely free of astigmatism, they seem to radiate the short lines that give them their so-called star shape. Swift movements of the eyes, which cause small but constant shifts of the lines upon the retina, create the illusion of twinkling. The radiating rays of street lights, headlights, or any other light seen in darkness, are also a result of our astigmatism.

Astigmatism that requires constant correction may cause severe headaches, due to the strain upon our focusing mechanisms. Such headaches are usually felt in the front of the head, although sometimes the entire head seems to pain. Fatigue and irritability are other symptoms.

The Aging Eye 9

The process of aging is not at all well understood. Why or how we age, what biochemical mechanisms are responsible, are questions that remain to be fully answered, but certain events or consequences of aging are known.

The aging process appears to be an uneven one, with some aspects of our life systems affected sooner than others. When we stop growing, generally in our teens, one portion of the aging process has begun. About the time we reach puberty and are capable of reproducing ourselves, the rate at which our bodies make new cells begins to slow. With this another aspect of aging begins, since our bodies become decreasingly able to repair or replace overworked or damaged tissue.

YOUR SIGHT: FOLKLORE, FACT AND COMMON SENSE

As time passes, our circulation becomes less effective. Arteries gradually lose flexibility, the valves of the heart and veins decline in efficiency, and the blood itself may no longer function at peak capacity in its dual role as a conveyor of essential chemicals and nutrients to the tissues and remover of metabolic wastes. Similarly, the other organs of the body, the kidneys, lungs, gastrointestinal tract, become more subject to stress, infection, and general debility.

Since each organ has an effect upon other organs, the effects of aging spread through the entire body. The glandular situation changes, nervous responses are neither as swift nor as precise, metabolic activity slows. Meanwhile, muscle tone and activity decline, hearing becomes less acute, and the eyes begin to lose their visual sharpness.

The gradual but inexorable blunting of eyesight with increasing age is a direct result of changes in muscle efficiency. This, in turn, affects the ability of the lens to accommodate for near and distant vision.

In a camera, accommodation is accomplished by moving the lens backward and forward, so that the sharpest possible picture will be focused on the film. This kind of movement is impossible in the human eye, as the crystalline lens always maintains the same distance from the retina. Instead, the lens adjusts to differing distances by varying the curve of its convex surface, thus increasing or decreasing its power.

The crystalline lens is an elastic body that is enclosed and slightly compressed by a capsule of tough, transparent membrane. When we look at a distant object, the capsule is pulled tight by the ciliary muscles, flattening the lens somewhat so that its curve is not as great and light is brought into focus upon the retina. When the eye turns to a closer object, the tension on the capsule is reduced, allowing the lens to spring back to a more convex or curved state, and bringing the light from the near object into focus.

The ring-shaped, muscular iris, lying just in front of the lens, opens or closes to change the size of the pupil, through which light passes to the lens. The opening or narrowing of the pupil is also related to the distance of the objects being viewed. When we look at something nearby our pupils contract; when we look at something off in the distance, they expand.

Pupil size also changes with emotional states, becoming smaller with anger, larger with fear. Pain also makes the pupils expand, while certain narcotics make them contract to the size of pinpoints.

Presbyopia

With age, the ability of the lenses to spring back to their fullest curve diminishes, and as this flexibility lessens, the ability to see close objects clearly declines. The name for this condition is *presbyopia*, "old man's eye."

When we are very young, we can usually see clearly objects held only an inch or two from our eyes. That is why the very finest embroidery and engraving in the Orient was done by children, and also in the West years ago. With each passing year, almost imperceptibly, the closest point of clear vision moves further away from us. At the same time, the muscles controlling the aperture of the iris slowly weaken, and the pupils gradually become smaller. The amount of light entering our eyes is steadily reduced, so that they require increasing amounts of light each passing year.

As a rule these changes are so gradual, and our ability to adjust to them so great, that they do not become troublesome until we reach the age of about forty. The newspaper we once read comfortably twelve or fourteen inches from our eyes now is blurred unless it is at least eighteen inches away. The dim light that was good enough for younger eyes becomes insufficient to read by. Finally we reach a point where reading and other close-up use of the eyes becomes distinctly uncomfortable. After hours of working or reading, we may experience eye fatigue and headaches, particularly in the area over the eyes. A visit to an ophthalmologist or an optometrist is past due.

Tall people, or at least people with long arms, require help somewhat later than those with shorter arms. The man with the longer arms can still hold the newspaper and other visual material further away, while the man with the shorter arms has used up all the available distance.

If the eyes have been free of astigmatism, hyperopia, or myopia when presbyopia develops, reading glasses will probably suffice to compensate for the changes in sight, and bring the near point of sharp vision close enough to permit us to read and do close work comfortably once more. These glasses will make distant objects appear blurred, however. Using reading glasses for anything other than close seeing is very uncomfortable. Unless other visual disorders are present, we can see perfectly well without glasses at middle and far distances.

The process of aging continues, unfortunately, beyond the need for the first pair of reading glasses. As the lenses continue to lose flexibility, near vision progressively deteriorates, and we find that even with reading glasses we are once more holding objects at arm's length.

The eyes should be examined regularly each year so that glasses can be corrected to adjust for changing vision. At about fifty, most people's amplitude of vision — the range of clear seeing between the nearest and furthest limits — will have narrowed to a point where they need correction for middle and distant vision as well as close. The majority of people with presbyopia ultimately come to need bifocal glasses, which are the equivalent of two sets

THE AGING EYE

of lenses in one frame; the lower set for close vision and the upper for distance.

By the age of about seventy, the ciliary muscles no longer have any significant effect upon the shape of the lens. Near vision will stabilize at that point, and will need no further correction. Until that time, the degree of change is so regular and inexorable that the ophthalmologist or optometrist can predict with remarkable accuracy just how much correction will be needed from year to year.

With increasing age there is a growing vulnerability to certain disease states that may affect vision. Glaucoma and cataracts have an increasing incidence with age. Diseases primarily affecting other parts of the body often also involve the eyes, including high blood pressure, diabetes, liver disease, kidney disease, and a number of infections, as well as glandular and nutritional disturbances.

Regular medical and eye examinations will not prevent disease or the changes that come with aging, but it is foolish to neglect such examinations. Many diseases can be prevented, and the damaging effects of others can be minimized or controlled by early diagnosis and prompt treatment. Glaucoma, for instance, need not cause blindness if detected and treated in time. Untreated, it can and usually does produce blindness. Nor need cataracts result in blindness.

After the age of forty we should have regular physical examinations every year and professional eye examinations for possible disease at least once every two years. Eye examinations for vision correction and eyeglass changes, of course, will be more frequent. Unlike wine, eyesight cannot be expected to improve with age.

10 Strabismus and Amblyopia: Deviated and Weakened Eyes

Crossed eyes, and other forms of strabismus, do not correct themselves. It is very important to realize that if we mistakenly wait for self-correction, some of the damage may become permanent. Perhaps two people out of a hundred have strabismus in some form, and in practically every case it can be corrected painlessly, without hazard, and with no loss of vision, if attended to early enough. If neglected, the eyes can still be aligned, but the damage done to the eyesight can rarely be fully reversed.

STRABISMUS AND AMBLYOPIA: DEVIATED AND WEAKENED EYES

A newborn infant has an innate tendency, but not the ability, to coordinate his eyes so that they both turn directly toward the object he is observing. The ability to coordinate usually becomes firmly established within a few months after birth. With such coordination, the infant then has the same image focused sharply on the fovea of each retina, and both images are combined to give a clear, unified, three-dimensional picture. This is called *binocular single vision* or *binocular fusion,* and it helps us judge both depth and distance.

If the two eyes do not line up, however, each retina has a different image focused upon it. This situation, in which the person sees a double image, is common to strabismus. It is known as *diplopia,* and it can be very disturbing. Not only does each eye look in a different direction, seeing a different object, but depth and distance perception are disturbed as well.

Strabismus can take a number of forms, depending upon which of the six muscles controlling the movement of each eye are involved. In *estropia,* one or both eyes may turn in; in *extropia,* or "walleyes," they may turn out. A relatively uncommon form of strabismus turns the eyes out of vertical alignment, one eye turned up or down while the other eye looks straight ahead.

Some strabismus is intermittent, the abnormality appearing only under conditions of illness, extreme fatigue, or emotional disturbance. It may also occur when muscle control is lost. The wall-eyed drunk is a person who, under the influence of alcohol, temporarily loses control of his eye muscles.

For the most part, however, strabismus begins in childhood, when it can be corrected most easily and generally with no damage. Nature itself makes an effort to compensate for strabismus. Since double vision is very disturbing to the brain it automatically begins to suppress the image of one eye, generally the eye that is off center. This suppression develops very quickly in a child, more slowly in an adult. Some adults with acquired strabismus are never able to rid themselves of the double image.

Under the circumstances it might appear that this image inhibition is a good thing. The brain, by refusing to accept visual data from one eye, presents the person with strabismus with a single rather than a double image. But it does it at the cost of the suppressed eye, for that eye is, for all practical purposes, blind. While diplopia is eliminated, the image that remains has all the characteristics of one seen by a person with a single effective eye. In addition to a loss of depth perception, there is a reduced ability to judge distance.

There is nothing wrong with the suppressed eye's ability to see at the onset of strabismus. But as time passes its acuity becomes less and less. This loss of visual acuity is known as *suppression amblyopia*. Tests taken of an eye before or even for a short while after strabismus develops show no loss of visual acuity that could be related to the deviation of the eye. But once suppression has occurred, tests show a deterioration in vision that may become so extreme that the affected eye can barely perceive light.

This kind of natural compensation for strabismus would be acceptable if the strabismus itself could not be corrected. But since the condition is correctable, especially in children, suppression amblyopia can become a definite liability. And the longer it exists, the more difficult correction becomes.

Treating Strabismus

The treatment begins with a thorough physical exmination by a doctor, and a check of the family history. It is important to know if any family traits are involved, whether any disease might be causing the condition, and to ascertain the general state of the patient's health.

After this general physical study, the ophthalmologist carefully examines the eyes to determine which eye is out of alignment and to what degree, and the precise state of the patient's vision. Such examinations are undergone by children and even infants. Thanks to sensitive modern instruments, the common belief that infants cannot have their eyes examined is simply no longer true.

Most cases of strabismus involve only one eye, the *deviated eye*. The uncrossed eye gradually takes over the major load of seeing. This process is called *fixation*. If it continues for any length of time, the deviated eye loses its visual acuity and develops suppression amblyopia.

Infants and small children will usually be treated with *occlusion therapy*. It is very simple; the good eye is covered with an eyepatch and the crossed eye is used exclusively. This is like strengthening a weak muscle by exercising it, and the result is generally successful.

Older children generally receive special eyeglasses that will help straighten the deviating eye. Regular examinations determine how well the correction is proceeding and whether new glasses are necessary.

After the eyes have remained straight for a period of several years, the glasses may be modified in strength. Often patients will be able to do without glasses for considerable periods, but the chances are that glasses will be necessary most of the time.

Should the eyes continue to remain crossed despite periodic changes of special eyeglasses and occlusion therapy, one or more operations may be necessary to correct the orbital muscles. These operations have practically no danger associated with them, but they may have to be repeated until the precise adjustment is made to straighten the eye.

Amblyopia — The Weakened Eye

According to Dr. Gunter K. von Noorden, associate professor of ophthalmology at Johns Hopkins University, about two million

Americans are affected by *amblyopia*. This word, derived from the Greek, means weak or dull vision, usually referring to conditions that cause a reduction in vision despite the fact that no known eye disease, past or present, is involved.

There are two main types of amblyopia. The less frequent type develops when the retina is not stimulated enough during infancy. The human eye is rarely injured by use or "excessive" use; it can definitely be harmed by not being used enough. An infant kept in a darkened room, with not enough toys or moving objects to engage its developing vision, is likely to develop amblyopia.

Another cause of this type of amblyopia may be an infantile cataract. This results in a cloudy or opaque lens, which prevents adequate light from stimulating the retina. Light to the retina can also be impeded by an opaque cornea, which may be due to infection or heredity. If these conditions are not corrected in time for the retina to "learn" to respond properly to light stimuli, then permanent damage may be done to the child's vision.

The second, more common form of amblyopia is the formation of images on each retina that are so unequal or confused that they cannot be combined by the brain into a single image. This second type of amblyopia is generally due to one of two forms of interference with normal fusion of the images we see with each eye; strabismus, resulting from an imbalance of the eye muscles, and *anisometropia*, which means "not having the same size." Anisometropia occurs when the focusing power of the two eyes is different, or when the same image is seen in two different sizes. Such a condition can result from marked variations in curvature of the corneas of each eye, differences in eyeball length, or the removal of a lens due to cataract.

In anisometropia, as in strabismus, the unequal images become too confusing for the brain to handle, so the image from one eye is suppressed. The suppressed eye then steadily loses its visual acuity and may be permanently impaired.

Until the last decade it was commonly believed that when amblyopia in a child continued beyond the sixth or seventh year it could not be reversed. Before that age, occlusion treatment was generally successful in correcting the condition.

The work of Drs. Alfred Bangerter of Switzerland and Kurt Cüppers of Germany has brought about a profound change in our understanding of amblyopia and its treatment. The two Europeans found that in amblyopia not only was there a decline in visual acuity, but the foveal area of the retina, where vision was sharpest, might shift to another place, leaving a blind spot where the fovea was normally located. This helped explain why occlusion therapy, which ordinarily corrected dim vision in amblyopia, was not effective in all cases, especially when the condition was of long standing.

To deal with this second factor in amblyopia the doctors introduced a variety of exercises and conditioning methods designed to retrain the eye so that the fovea could become useful once again. This approach is known as *pleoptic therapy,* and has been widely applied in many parts of the world. Pleoptic therapy does not work in all cases, but it does help a number of children whose amblyopia has existed too long to be corrected by occlusion therapy. In many instances, according to Dr. Goodwin M. Breinin of New York University, it can help improve the visual acuity of adults as well.

Thanks to these new advances, amblyopic children past the age of six or seven need not be considered permanently impaired, but early detection and treatment remain the best insurance against permanent damage.

Alcohol and "Seeing Double"

The damaging effect of even a single ounce of alcoholic beverage upon vision has been demonstrated in a number of tests. At Yale University some years ago it was shown that there was a

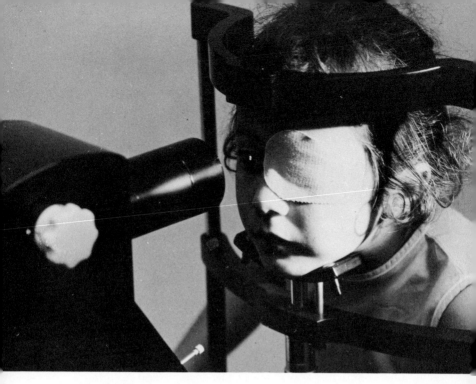

Fundus fixation photography of interior of eye of young patient with amblyopia. University of Miami, Florida.

An amblyopic patient with strabismus is examined with a major amblyoscope at Tulane University.

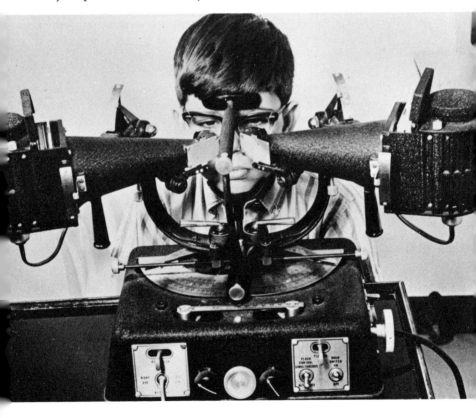

diminution of peripheral vision with the very first drink. This effect is transient, ceasing when the alcohol and its metabolic by-products leave the system. In 1965, a test was conducted in the Hamburg General Hospital in Germany by Dr. Hans Gert Zuschlag to check the effect of alcohol upon binocular fusion — the combination of the images received by both eyes into a single picture.

In the test, twenty-six volunteers were subjected to six different examinations before and after taking considerable amounts of alcohol. It was found that when the level of alcohol in the blood was greater than 0.7 percent, every one of the volunteers showed some impairment of vision. In twenty-three of these persons, the impairment of vision was considerable, with a marked reduction in their ability to fuse the two images.

Dr. Zuschlag also found that most of the volunteers, in addition to seeing double, showed a tendency to either crossed or walleyes while intoxicated; and eleven of them had damaged stereoscopic vision with a corresponding loss of depth and distance vision.

Glaucoma 11

Despite the fact that early treatment can stop its more damaging ravages, glaucoma still remains responsible for about one case of blindness in every seven. Most such blindness is unnecessary. Those who go blind from glaucoma are usually as much victims of ignorance or apathy as of the disease. By failing to have regular eye examinations, which become increasingly important past the age of forty, and simply by being unable to recognize the signs of impending trouble, they condemn themselves to irreversible damage before the presence of disease is even suspected.

Quite often in this disease, central vision remains perfectly normal until blindness is imminent. For this reason, visual acuity tests do not help much in detecting the ailment. On the other hand, glaucoma can usually be detected very early in its course by a simple test of eye pressure. Once detected, glaucoma can often be kept under control by medical treatment, or in some cases by an operation.

Experts have estimated that as many as one million Americans over the age of forty have glaucoma today and *do not know it*. Men and women are equally susceptible. The disease usually involves both eyes, and seems to occur more often in farsighted people than in nearsighted. There is a congenital form of glaucoma that affects children, but it is chiefly a disease of the middle and later years. It is rare between the ages of ten and twenty and after seventy.

In glaucoma, the eyeball may be likened to a basketball that constantly has air pumped into it but does not have a safety valve to allow excess air to escape. Increased pressure in glaucoma is caused by the aqueous humor, the waterlike fluid that fills the space between the front of the eye and lens. This fluid enters the eye through the ciliary body, a circular organ located behind the iris, and helps maintain the proper outward pressure in order that, among other things, the eye keeps its shape and the cornea keeps its proper curve, so that light can enter the eye with a minimum of distortion.

If the internal pressure is to remain constant, the fluid must be able to leave the eye at the same rate that it enters. Normally, this is what does happen. The fluid circulates through the eye, is filtered through a layer of porous fibers called the *trabecula*, which acts very much like the sieve in a kitchen sink, and passes out of the eye through a circular channel called the *Canal of Schlemm*.

But if the aqueous humor enters the eye at a faster rate than it leaves, pressure builds up, causing glaucoma. This unusual pressure slowly deforms the optic nerve, which gradually takes the shape of a deepening cup. The field of vision diminishes as cupping becomes more extreme, but since the macula lutea — the area of sharp vision — is often the last part of the optic nerve to be affected, central vision often remains normal for a considerable time.

Scientists have known about glaucoma for generations — Hippocrates referred to it some twenty-five hundred years ago — but it was not until the last century that eye specialists were finally able to describe what happens in this disease and to develop appropriate treatment for it. The reason for the increase in pressure appears to be some obstruction that interferes with the exit of the fluid from the eye, rather than any change in the nature of the fluid or increase in its production.

The most common type of glaucoma, as well as the most destructive, is *primary glaucoma*. This, in turn, is divided into *acute congestive (angle block) glaucoma* and *chronic (wide angle) simple glaucoma*.

Another type of glaucoma is congenital, due to a genetic predisposition or to a malformation that impedes the draining of aqueous fluid from the eye. Finally there is *secondary glaucoma*, the cause of which rests with some other disease or disorder that may produce obstruction of the eye's drainage system.

Ordinarily, primary glaucoma takes a considerable time to develop. Acute congestive glaucoma, however, often causes so sudden an increase in pressure that swift emergency measures are needed. Some people are highly susceptible to acute congestive glaucoma. The opening of the iris with its consequent dilation of the pupil, can cause an obstruction of the drainage system and result in an acute attack of glaucoma. For such people, anything that might cause the pupils to dilate widely can be dangerous. Strong emotion, pain, the use of certain drugs, watching television or motion pictures in a darkened room, or even stargazing on a moonless night might trigger an attack.

Certain clues point to the possibility of acute congestive

glaucoma. In mild attacks, the appearance of rainbows or halos around lights, as well as some discomfort or pain in the eyes, are telltale signs. If these symptoms occur in the dark or in dim light, during television-watching for instance, and subside during sleep, the likelihood of glaucoma is increased.

In more severe attacks, the pain in the eye is intense and may be accompanied by headache, nausea, and even vomiting. Vision may be blurred; the eye may be red and the cornea appear hazy.

Any of these signs demands an immediate appointment with a physician or opthalmologist. Prompt diagnosis and treatment can be sight-saving.

The onset of chronic glaucoma is not at all dramatic. It may develop insidiously, without noticeable symptoms, over a period of years. There may be a gradual appearance of halos around light, plus a progressive diminution of the field of vision until most of the peripheral vision is gone. If the process continues too long, loss of sight may be complete. No one should wait for symptoms to appear before visiting an eye doctor.

Dr. Harold G. Scheie, professor of ophthalmology at the University of Pennsylvania, gives this warning: "The prevention of blindness from glaucoma will be possible only with periodic ocular examinations at least once every two years, and with constant vigilance on the part of an informed medical profession."

Ironically, although chronic simple glaucoma is called "simple," its diagnosis is extremely difficult. Regular tests for the condition should begin at thirty-five, and are essential at forty. Since patients with chronic simple glaucoma usually have no symptoms early in the disease except for some occasional blurred vision, headache, or a feeling of fullness in the eye, the physician or ophthalmologist must test for this disease regularly, even in the absence of any symptoms.

With a specially made contact lens called a *goniscope*, the physician examines the forward chamber of the eye to see whether the base of the iris blocks or is likely to block the exit of aqueous fluid through the Canal of Schlemm.

Another test makes use of the *ophthalmoscope,* a device invented in 1851 by the great German scientist Hermann von Helmholtz. The ophthalmoscope focuses a beam of light into the eye and magnifies the reflection. This instrument has made it possible to examine the interior of the living eye and study in detail the various parts, including the retina and optic nerve. The ophthalmoscope may show very early cupping of the optic nerve, a sign of the disease that may exist long before actual symptoms appear.

Finally, the doctor can test the internal pressure of the eye. If he has a very sensitive touch and a great amount of experience he can do this with his fingertips, pressing gently through the eyelid. More accurate, and certainly more practical, is the *tonometer,* one of the most important instruments used in the detection of glaucoma. The doctor first administers a drop or so of anesthetic, then places the tonometer upon the cornea and measures the pressure exerted upon it from the interior of the eye. The higher the reading on the scale of the tonometer, the lower the pressure inside the eye.

When a physician suspects the presence of glaucoma but cannot prove it by conventional means, he might use what is known as a *provocative test* to provoke symptoms. The patient drinks over a quart of water within a five-minute period. Every fifteen minutes for the next hour and a half, the pressure inside the eye is tested with the tonometer. Because the system is now flooded with water which spreads throughout the body, the amount of fluid entering the eye will increase, and if there is any interference with the rate at which this fluid leaves the eye, pressure will rise. This test often discloses glaucoma in difficult cases, but it is not foolproof; it may show a negative result, even though glaucoma is present. Whenever there is any doubt at all, the complete examination should be repeated within three to six months.

According to recent surveys, one person in every forty past the age of forty has glaucoma. Failure to detect and treat this condition in time leads to blindness, and this grim result *can* be prevented.

Treating Glaucoma to Prevent Blindness

The heart of the problem in treating glaucoma is finding an effective way of permitting the aqueous fluid to leave the eye at the same rate that it enters. This means relieving the obstruction that is impeding the outflow.

A person with chronic simple glaucoma will take certain drugs known as *miotics.* Miotic drugs, usually administered as eyedrops, close down the iris and contract the pupil, in many cases thereby reducing the obstruction caused by the pressure of the wide-open iris against the drainage area.

Other drugs are also used, some by injection and others by mouth. Some are intended to relieve the obstruction, and others are used to reduce the amount of aqueous fluid secreted into the eye by the ciliary body.

If medical treatment does not succeed in reducing the abnormal pressure, the next resort is surgery. The most effective operation is designed to create an artificial passageway, known as a *fistula,* through the outer wall of the eye, so that the fluid can leave the interior and drain into the subconjunctival space. Fistula operations are not easy, and may be accompanied by complications.

Acute congestive glaucoma does not respond well to medication, except occasionally in its very early stages. The main problem with this type of glaucoma is that the drainage space at the base of the iris is confined within an abnormally narrow angle formed by the iris and cornea. (This problem gives the disease its other

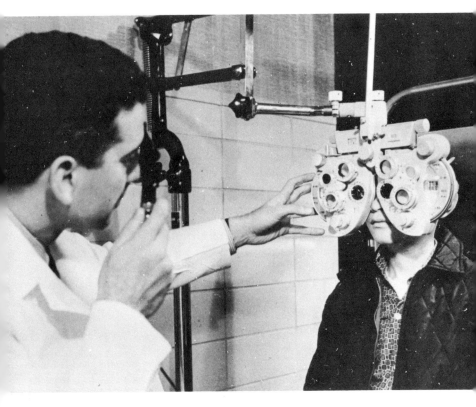

Scientist at Albert Einstein College of Medicine examines eyes of a young diabetic patient, in a study to determine the relationship of diabetes to glaucoma.

name, *angle block glaucoma*.) Miotic drugs do not relieve the obstruction effectively, so the ophthalmologist must perform a *peripheral iridectomy,* an operation in which a tiny bit of iris is removed to allow the aqueous humor to flow through from front to back.

If performed early enough, the iridectomy also prevents the iris from coming into contact with the drainage area — the *trabecula* — and obstructing it. This operation usually cures the glaucoma, and is accompanied by few complications; but unfortunately, if the acute attack of glaucoma has continued more than a day or two, or if the iris adheres to the trabecula as a result of repeated attacks, an iridectomy will not succeed. In such cases the surgeon must resort to the fistula operation that is performed for medically untreatable chronic glaucoma. The advantages of an early diagnosis, which would permit the simpler, less dangerous operation, are obvious.

Thanks to the German von Helmholtz, who invented the ophthalmoscope; the Norwegian Hjalmar Schiotz, who made the tonometer; the Frenchman Louis Laqueur, who pioneered the use of miotic drugs; the German Albrecht von Graefe and the Englishman Priestly Smith, who developed the surgical procedures; and the other scientists who have helped pave the way, the ancient scourge of glaucoma has been brought under control. The fact that glaucoma can be treated so that its damage is stopped and blindness prevented represents one of the great advances of modern healing. Yet because of ignorance and neglect, much glaucoma remains undetected, and thousands of unfortunate people are doomed to tragically unnecessary loss of sight.

Cataract: A Curtain Against Light   12

Thousands of years ago, in Egypt and then in Greece and Rome, cataract was recognized as a defect of the lens, which for some unknown reason became opaque and acted as a curtain against light. Early surgeons performed an operation called *couching* — pushing the crystalline lens out of the way with a needle inserted through the cornea. The lens remained inside the eye, but because it was out of the line of sight between the pupil and retina, it did not interfere with the passage of light. Many such operations were successful, and the patients frequently recovered some sight. In his book on surgery, the *Susruta-Samhita,* which has been described as one of the major treasures of human heritage, the pre-Christian Indian physician Susruta not only outlined the different types of cataract, but also described a technique for their treatment.

Similar operations were performed by more primitive people in the Pacific islands, and by the pre-Columbian Indians of the Andean highlands. This might lead us to question why, when effective cataract surgery has existed for thousands of years, there was no equally effective treatment for glaucoma. The answer lies in the act of recognition. Primitive healers could develop relatively effective treatments for ailments whose nature and cause they could recognize. They could treat wounds, cuts, and bruises, whose origins they knew, with poultices and early pain killers, such as poppy juice or infusions of willow bark (a substance, incidentally, chemically similar to aspirin). But when they were faced with infections or internal diseases whose causes were not apparent, they were less effective as doctors.

They attributed these less obvious ailments to magical spells, infestations of demons, or the anger of the gods, and treated them by efforts to lift the spells, drive out the demons, or placate the gods. In a high percentage of cases this approach was even associated with cures. After all, much illness runs its course and then vanishes, regardless of whether or not the patient is given good medical treatment, innocuous medical treatment, magical treatment, faith healing, or no treatment at all.

Early physicians developed a rational treatment for cataract because they were able to see a rational cause. In most cases the lens of the eye became opaque, and this was invariably related to a diminution of vision. It followed, then, that if the opaque portion of the eye could somehow be gotten rid of or pushed aside, sight would be restored.

The problem with glaucoma was quite different. There were

no obvious signs that could be recognized and dealt with directly. Instead there was pain, some headache — then blindness. Clearly, to the early physicians, this was a matter of demons, gods, or witches.

In cataract there is a partial or complete clouding of the lens. It is the lens itself that becomes cloudy or opaque — no strange growth is involved, nor does a film form over the lens, as many people believe. Just what mechanism is involved in making the lens turn cloudy is not at all clear, although there are a number of reasonable explanations.

The crystalline lens is a structure of tightly packed cells. These cells consist mainly of protein. Ordinarily the lens proteins are transparent, like the proteins in an egg white. In the cataractous lens, however, there is a progressive coagulation and opacification of lens protein, roughly as the transparent egg-white protein coagulates and becomes opaque when cooked.

Some cataracts cover only a small portion of the lens, and either stop progressing or progress so slowly that loss of vision remains relatively minor. Other cataracts may continue to develop until the whole lens becomes opaque and blindness results. When this point is reached, the cataract is said to be *mature*. The blindness of cataract is not an absolute blackout, but a thickening fog through which, in time, only strong light can penetrate as a hazy glow.

There are various types of cataract, distinguished by their appearance and other characteristics in addition to the rate of their development.

The most common type has no detectable cause other than the attrition of the aging process. This is called *senile cataract,* but it is not necessarily associated with senility; it may begin to develop in the fifties, or even earlier. Some scientists suggest that, while genetic predisposition may have a part in senile cataract formation, the direct factor is the accumulation over the years of damage done by exposure of the eye to ultraviolet radiation of sunlight, as well as the thermal effect of infrared light.

Congenital cataract, however, may be present at birth. Often this type of cataract is hereditary, but sometimes it is caused by an infection in the mother early in pregnancy. German measles, along with a number of other infections, can be an important cause of childhood cataracts.

Traumatic cataracts are the result of injuries to the lens, and may appear almost immediately after the event or many months later. The injury has to penetrate the lens capsule and permit the entry of aqueous humor into the lens itself to cause a cataract.

Cataracts can also be caused by intense heat, and occur with a fairly high degree of frequency among glassblowers and steelworkers. Exposure to various forms of nuclear radiation, such as X rays and subatomic particles, may also cause cataracts. For a time such cataracts were relatively common among nuclear scientists, but with adequate precautions they have now become rare.

Secondary cataracts are by-products of other diseases, such as iritis, glaucoma, detached retina, various eye tumors, and hemorrhages. Another type of secondary cataract is the *metabolic cataract,* the most common of which is the *sugar cataract* of diabetes. Dr. V. Everett Kinsey, professor of ophthalmology at Wayne State University in Detroit, has produced cataracts in experimental animals by feeding them *xylose,* a form of sugar. His research into the biochemical steps that apparently lead to cataract formation are of particular interest, since they suggest the possibility of future medical treatment. (See Chapter 27.)

Certain drugs and chemicals can also produce lens opacities, known as *toxic cataracts.* When taken into the body, ergot, certain heavy metals, cortisone drugs, and other substances seem to interfere with the normal biochemical processes, perhaps blocking the activity of certain enzymes, and causing the deterioration of the lens proteins.

Whatever the type of cataract and whatever the initial cause, they all meet at a single focal point — the breakdown and opacification of the protein in the crystalline lens. Could the process somehow be stopped before that point, it might be possible to prevent cataract formation.

With modern surgical treatment, about ninety-eight of every one hundred cataracts can be prevented from causing blindness; and yet, according to a recent estimate of the U.S. Public Health Service, cataracts have been responsible for about one-fourth of the blindness in this country. Like the statistics about glaucoma, this is particularly tragic because it is unnecessary.

Treatment of Cataract

For thousands of years the couching operation remained the sole effective rational treatment for cataract.

Of course, there were and are less rational treatments. In the Missouri hill country the tail of a black cat, drawn daily across the affected eye, is believed to be a cure for a cataract. Other magical and superstitious "cures" involve various forms of witchcraft, incantation, and prayer, as well as pilgrimages to religious shrines. Occasionally these methods have appeared effective, relieving blindness resulting from certain hysterical states, but they could never have restored clarity to a lens made opaque by a cataract.

Even the couching operation came into considerable disrepute in Europe for a time. The rational medicine of the Greeks and Arabs was considered heretical and a challenge to the religious medicine of the early church, which sought to achieve curative miracles by faith, prayer, and the laying on of hands. Another factor was poor sanitation. While the Egyptian, Hindu, and Arab surgeons maintained clear professional standards and had some concept of the need for cleanliness, this was not at all true of Europeans.

The high quality of Eastern surgery was certainly indicated by the writings of the Persian, Ibn Sina, known to the Western world as Avicenna. In the fifth volume of his great work on medicine and surgery, the *Canon,* Ibn Sina described the couching operation in meticulous detail. Toward the close of the eleventh century, reports of this operation for cataract were brought back to Europe, where it came to be performed by a horde of untrained and unskilled practitioners, rather than by physicians.

There was an interesting reason for this, dating back to a concept inherited from early Greece. Despite its traditional democracy, which was confined to Greek citizens, Greece was a slave state. All labor was done by slaves, and the Greek citizens were thus freed to indulge their minds in philosophy, poetry, scientific speculations, and other matters. The free Greeks could and did become physicians, talking to patients, examining them, diagnosing disease and prescribing treatment. Surgery, which at the very least required cutting and lancing, was manual labor, fit only for slaves.

To this very day in Great Britain, physicians carry the title of doctor but surgeons are called "mister." In medieval Europe, those who performed any surgery, including the operation for cataract, were considered mere laborers by the medical profession. It was because of these peculiar circumstances that the early barbers, skilled in the use of razors and other cutting instruments, began to be called upon to do bloodletting and boil lancing, finally evolving into barber-surgeons.

Against this background, it can easily be seen why the couching operation, which was widely performed in Europe following the First Crusade, almost invariably failed. Not only was the affected eye usually lost, but frequently serious additional damage was done by infection. Inevitability of infection was as much a part of the times as low quality of surgery.

During this period in Europe's history cleanliness was believed closer to heresy than to godliness. Mortification of the flesh and living in "holy" dirt were associated with saintliness and virtue. Nevertheless as more civilized concepts came to Europe better surgical procedures gradually evolved, and relative cleanliness during an operation became increasingly acceptable. The couching operation continued to be performed, with a better degree of success.

The first actual removal of a cataractous lens occurred as the result of a surgical accident.

Toward the end of the sixteenth century, a German barber-surgeon named George Bartisch, who became the oculist to August, Elector of Saxony, devised a variation of the couching operation. Instead of inserting a needle through the front of the eye and pushing the lens back, Bartisch introduced the needle through the side of the eye, behind the cornea. He then cut open the capsule containing the lens and pushed the lens down to the floor of the eye.

Occasionally, unless extreme care was exercised in placing the needle correctly, the lens would be pushed forward against the iris instead of backward and down. Since the iris is a very delicate structure, pressure from a displaced lens could cause it serious damage. Following such an accident in 1688, a barber-surgeon named Stephen Blaukaart removed the displaced lens through a small incision he made in the cornea for that purpose. As far as is known, this was the first time that the lens was actually removed from the eye in an operation for cataract.

Later, Jacques Daviel made lens removal a standard approach to the treatment of cataract. By the time Daviel died in 1762, he had reportedly removed 434 opaque lenses from cataract patients, and had succeeded in restoring vision to more than 380 of them.

Couching had finally been replaced by a more effective surgical approach.

This operation was further improved by Albertus von Graefe in the middle of the nineteenth century. The noted surgeon added the removal of a small section of the iris — *iridectomy,* also used in the surgical treatment of glaucoma — to the lens extraction. This saved the iris as a whole from the damage that could occur because of the cataract operation.

After this modification by von Graefe, who reported 95 percent success in a lifetime total of some nine hundred cataract operations, very little change took place in the procedure up to the present day. In recent years, although the operation remains essentially the same, a number of technical improvements have made cataract surgery safer and more satisfactory. Instruments are better, and the recently developed practice of performing the operation under microscopic control is a great step forward. The use of an enzyme, *alpha chymotrypsin,* has made it easier to free the cataract from its attachments, thus simplifying the operation.

"During the last few years rapid freezing has been introduced as another means of taking hold of the cataract to get it out of the eye, safely, surely, and gently," reports Dr. John M. McLean, professor of clinical surgery (ophthalmology) at Cornell University Medical College, "and this is only one of the recent advances in the surgical attack on a disease that we should learn to prevent, or, if it occurs, treat without operation."

Dr. McLean anticipates a time in the not-too-distant future when cataracts will be a medical rather than a surgical problem, preferably one of preventive medicine.

When the opaque lens is removed, the curtain that has descended over vision disappears. Light can once again enter through the pupil and pass through the eye to the retina, where it is converted to signals that are carried by the optic nerve to the brain. There is only one thing wrong — the light is not focused, because the lens is gone. Consequently, it is possible to distinguish objects and movement, but not details.

For this reason, after a healing period of at least two weeks following the operation, the ophthalmologist must provide a substitute lens. So far cataract glasses have not been able to return vision to normal, but, with adjustment of the lenses and considerable education of the patient, functional vision is restored.

Until recent times, cataract glasses were rather thick, heavy lenses worn as eyeglasses. Despite a number of improvements they remain somewhat inefficient. Contact lenses are a recent improvement in this area, and according to most specialists come much closer to restoring normal vision. Unfortunately they are not suitable for everyone, particularly the elderly. Nor can they be worn at all times.

Attempts are being made to implant a plastic lens inside the eye. If successful, this would certainly restore the total visual situation much closer to normal.

The present state of cataract treatment has been summed up by Dr. McLean as follows: "Cataracts can be handled by surgery with a very high prospect of success. We will continue to improve our surgical approaches and our optical rehabilitation but this is not the ultimate goal. That goal should be cataract prevention, if possible, and medical treatment where prevention is not possible. To achieve this, we must first learn not only why cataract occurs but how it occurs. This understanding of the details of cataract formation can only be obtained through intensive research."

13 The Detached Retina

Sudden flashes of light in the lower part of the visual field may be the first sign of the condition known as *retinal detachment*. Other signs may be showers of spots before the affected eye, a hazy or wavy "curtain" in front of the eye, or an unexplained decline in visual acuity.

Detachment of the retina is serious, but it is not as common a cause of blindness as cataract or glaucoma. With proper treatment it can almost always be cured.

The choroid layer contains the blood vessels that nourish the retina and its millions of nerves. If the retina peels away or separates from it, its essential blood supply will be reduced and it can no longer effectively do its job of "seeing." If the blood supply is cut off completely the retina becomes utterly useless, its nerves unable to convey patterns of visual impulses to the brain. At this stage, blindness ensues.

Whatever the immediate cause of retinal detachment, the condition is clearly more frequent in people over fifty years old. A recent survey at the Retina Service of the Massachusetts Eye and Ear Infirmary showed that of 451 patients with retinal detachment, 56 percent were over fifty. According to Dr. W. S. Duke-Elder, a world-renowned British specialist, detachment is most likely to occur between the ages of fifty and sixty, the decade when senile changes in the eye usually become apparent.

The aging factor indicates that retinal detachments, along with age-associated cataract and glaucoma, are bound to become more frequent as longevity increases. Many diseases common today were once relatively rare because we did not live long enough to contract them. It is one of the ironies of science that each year of increased life expectancy must, for the present at least, be paid for in increased vulnerability.

However, age is not the sole determining factor in retinal detachment. Drs. R. T. Smith and L. H. Pierce at the Massachusetts Eye and Ear Infirmary have found that approximately 22 percent of their patients had suffered from myopia. In them, retinal detachment developed earlier in life, especially if the myopia was serious.

Direct or indirect injury to the retina may also cause detachment. The indirect trauma might be difficult to evaluate, because an accident or disease may set into motion a complex chain of events, with retinal detachment a distant consequence.

Dr. P. Robb McDonald of the University of Pennsylvania observes that retinal detachment occurs more frequently in men than in women, in a 60 to 40 ratio. He suggests that this "can probably be explained by the greater exposure to trauma, direct or indirect, that the man is likely to encounter in his everyday activities."

Why the retina should come loose from the choroid layer of the eye, much as a moistened postage stamp peels away from an envelope, is not clear, but it is generally accepted that the process begins with some damage to the retina itself — a tear, break, or hole. This may be the result of a sharp blow to the eye, or it might be due to an inherited structural defect in the retina. Whatever the cause, a break in the retina occurs, but this alone is not enough to cause detachment.

Next, fluid seeps through the break, forcing its way behind the retina and separating it from the choroid, to which it is only loosely attached. The fluid comes from the vitreous body or humor, the jellylike substance that fills the eyeball's chamber between the lens and the retina. If the vitreous humor always kept its jellied consistency and provided no fluid, the retina would probably not become detached. However, for reasons that are not yet understood, the aging process seems to cause some liquefaction as well as shrinkage of the gel, making fluid available to float the retina away from the choroid.

Shrinkage of the vitreous can also cause retinal detachment. In some people, the gel may come to adhere strongly to the surface of the retina. Then, as the vitreous humor shrinks with age, it pulls the retina away from the choroid on the other side.

Most people with retinal detachment do not know what is wrong with them, beyond the fact that they are not seeing as clearly as before through the involved eye. The sudden flashes of light, the wavy curtain or the shower of spots, known as *vitreous opacities* or *floaters,* are only remembered after an examining physician asks about them. Had these early signs sent them to the ophthalmologist promptly, easier and more complete correction of the visual disturbance might have been possible, and serious detachment prevented.

Illustration of retinal detachment.

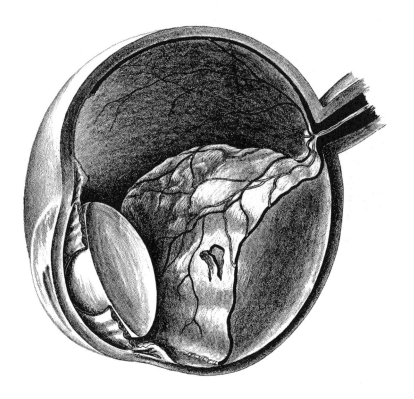

Circulation of the retina, demonstrated by use of fluorescein. The injected fluorescein shows aneurisms as well as a block of the retina's arterial circulation. This study was performed by Dr. James H. Allen, Department of Ophthalmology, Tulane University.

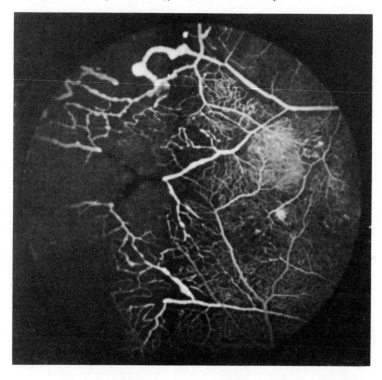

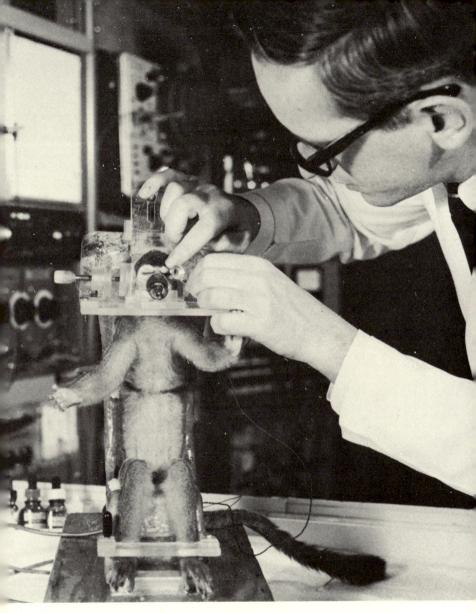

Dr. Alson E. Braley, of the University of Iowa, prepares to measure the retinal capability of a monkey by means of experimental electroretinogram (ERG).

Retinal detachment is usually diagnosed through the ophthalmoscope. This instrument not only detects the actual separation of the retina from the choroid, but also reveals the holes and tears that precede retinal detachment.

Naturally, the greater the degree of detachment, the easier it is to detect and the more difficult it is to achieve full correction. Dr. McDonald of the University of Pennsylvania comments: "Unfortunately, the diagnosis of any retinal detachment is frequently all too easy by the time the patient is first seen by the ophthalmologist. We would prefer to see the patients when the diagnosis would be more difficult, especially before macular vision is lost. The earlier a detachment is recognized and the less extensive it is, the better the prognosis for good vision."

Reattaching the Retina

In one case out of four, a person with a detached retina in one eye will develop the same problem in the other. It is therefore important to treat the first eye as soon as possible, and not rely on the remaining eye to carry the burden of vision indefinitely.

Prior to this century there was no effective way of treating the problem. In 1919 a Swiss physician, Jules Gonin, suggested that retinal detachment could be corrected by cauterizing the tear in the retina, thus causing an adhesive scar that would once more fix the retina to the choroid. Gonin had an opportunity to test his theory when an elderly woman who had been suffering for a number of years from retinal detachment began to fear, incorrectly, that the defect was somehow contagious and would affect the good eye. She hurried to Dr. Gonin and told him she wanted the defective eye removed.

Instead of taking out the eye, the Swiss ophthalmologist decided that neither his patient nor he had anything to lose if he first attempted to correct the detachment with *thermocautery*.

The attempt succeeded, and the modern era of retinal surgery opened.

Today Gonin's basic thesis is still applied, but techniques have improved considerably. The operation is usually performed under general anesthesia, and takes from one to four hours. The adhesive scar is made by electric diathermy, or by freezing. *Cryosurgery,* one of the latest developments in the treatment of retinal detachment, has several advantages over other forms of surgery, particularly in that it is less likely to cause damage to the vitreous than electric diathermy or the ultra-intense light known as the *laser beam.* The laser beam and another similar approach, *photocoagulation,* are useful in preventing detachments and treating them in their very early stages. Continuing research will produce further refinements and improvements, but Gonin's thermocautery has been able to correct retinal detachment and restore vision in at least seven out of ten cases.

Anyone who has had a retinal detachment would be wise to avoid activities that might produce sudden jars or falls, such as skiing, horseback riding, diving, or driving in heavy traffic where sudden stops might be necessary. He should also know that there are at present no drugs or medications that will prevent fluid-causing changes in the vitreous, or that will strengthen the retina.

14 Diabetic and Hypertensive Retinopathy

Retinopathy is simply any abnormal condition or disease of the retina that does not involve an inflammation. Generally, it refers to a degenerative change — a breakdown in the structure, the chemistry, or the circulation of the retina. Senile macular degeneration, a major cause of blindness, is a form of retinopathy associated with aging. Retinopathy is also frequently a by-product of one of two diseases that are increasing at an extremely rapid rate — diabetes and hypertension, or high blood pressure.

Diabetic Retinopathy

Some four million Americans are currently estimated to be suffering from diabetes, with two hundred thousand new cases diagnosed every year, and approximately forty-five thousand persons in the United States are blind as a result of this disease. The sugar cataract of diabetes accounts for some of these cases, but most were caused by retinopathy.

The investigation of diabetic retinopathy was long seriously handicapped because no animal could be found that developed it, but in 1962 it was noted that diabetic dogs developed retinopathy very similar to the early retinopathy seen in diabetic humans. This provided the first opportunity to study the serious eye ailment experimentally, and to test new methods of treatment.

The development of diabetic retinopathy is usually related to the length of time the patient has had diabetes. Studies by Dr. Arnall Patz of Johns Hopkins University School of Medicine suggest that retinopathy appears in about 70 percent of the people who have had diabetes for fifteen years. In those who have had diabetes for twenty-five years, approximately 90 to 95 percent have some degree of retinopathy.

For a number of years medical scientists have been trying to learn the process whereby diabetes, which has long been considered a disease of carbohydrate metabolism, could produce damage to the retina. Within the last few years it has become increasingly clear that diabetes involves the circulation and other body systems as much as it involves a defect in the ability to utilize sugars and starches. In diabetic retinopathy the major factor is circulatory — the diabetes somehow causes abnormalities, such as aneurysms, in the capillaries, the tiny vessels that deliver arterial blood to the retina and pick up waste products for removal through the veins.

Aneurysms are small balloonlike enlargements of the capillaries which are likely to burst and produce tiny hemorrhages. In 1960, Drs. David Cogan and Toichiro Kuwabara of the Howe Laboratory in Boston devised an ingenious technique for studying the cells in the walls of the retinal capillaries. They have been able to show that these cells undergo progressive damage in patients who are diabetic.

It would seem, from this and other research, that diabetics who undergo damage to the circulatory system suffer an interference with the delivery of needed oxygen and nutrients to the cells and nerves of the retina. Furthermore, the blood which normally delivers these products through the capillary walls is impeded from taking up and removing waste products.

Exactly how diabetes causes this damage to the retinal capillaries is not at all clear.

One theory suggests that *pituitary growth hormone,* secreted by the pituitary gland, is a factor in diabetic retinopathy, as well as in diabetes itself. In excessive amounts this hormone seems to be associated with diabetes in humans, and can also produce diabetes in dogs. Recently, scientists in both the United States and Canada have shown that when dogs become diabetic as a result of growth hormone administration, they often develop the same type of retinopathy found in naturally diabetic dogs.

Another theory proposes that diabetic retinopathy is linked to a defect in fat metabolism. People with diabetes appear not to utilize fats normally. One feature of the disease is a very rapid development of *atherosclerosis* — hardening of the blood vessels resulting from abnormal deposits of fat on the interior walls of the arteries.

Atherosclerosis, as we well know, is by no means confined to diabetics; it has become increasingly common in this country. But it occurs in diabetics in a much higher ratio than in nondiabetics;

in almost all diabetics, in fact, and in them it develops at an accelerated rate.

The atherosclerosis seen in diabetes can affect virtually all the blood vessels, inducing *vascular disease*. This may impede circulation to the extremities, and it can also result in damage to the circulation of the kidneys and eyes.

Fortunately, in many diabetics the retinal damage is minor, and has little if any effect upon vision. But where the retinopathy causes serious interference with vision and threatens blindness, treatment becomes very important; and for most cases of diabetic retinopathy there is no generally accepted form of therapy.

One approach has had promising results in a number of selected cases. The operation is called *hypophysectomy,* and involves the removal of all or part of the pituitary gland. Various forms of this operation have not only checked the advance of the retinopathy but have even resulted in some restoration of lost vision. Several successes of this type were reported in 1966 by Dr. C. A. Fager of the Lahey Clinic in Boston and Drs. S. B. Reese and R. F. Bradley of Boston's Joslin Clinic.

Another approach to the treatment of diabetic retinopathy makes use of *photocoagulation,* one of the methods applied to retinal detachment. Intense light from a special lamp using a xenon arc is focused on the retina, and destroys some of the blood vessels and aneurysms. This treatment does damage of its own, but it is believed to prevent and limit some of the more serious damage caused by retinopathy. Drs. Paul C. Wetzig and C. Neal Jepson of the Colorado Springs Eye Clinic have treated more than one hundred and eleven eyes in this fashion. In the seventy-five cases that they followed for from three to five years, they reported "good evidence that the progress of the diabetic lesion may be slowed."

While hypophysectomy has produced good results in some patients, and photocoagulation may prove to be of benefit, both approaches to diabetic retinopathy are extreme and could certainly not be recommended in every case. Hypophysectomy, for instance, can have far-reaching effects upon the system. The removal of the pituitary, the gland that controls the operation of the other glands in the body, means serious changes. Some of the hormones ordinarily produced by this gland have been synthesized and can be administered, but a number of important hormones will be missing.

In a noted Eastern center for the treatment of diabetics, a young woman, recently married, was threatened with blindness resulting from retinopathy. At the same time, she was desperately anxious to have a child. This posed her physician a heartbreaking dilemma. The hypophysectomy would probably save her sight, but would almost certainly destroy her chances of conceiving. On the other hand, the excessive amounts of growth hormone produced during pregnancy, plus the stress of childbearing, would make blindness inevitable.

Fortunately, such decisions do not have to be faced every day.

There has been much controversy as to whether good medical control of diabetes will in any way affect the progress of associated retinopathy. The available evidence appears to suggest that ocular damage takes an independent course. This is a gloomy conclusion, but the outlook has been brightened considerably by reports from research centers in England and the United States regarding a drug that may have a beneficial effect in diabetic retinopathy. (This drug, it must be emphasized, may not prove as beneficial as early tests indicated. Enough drugs have failed after showing early experimental promise to pave a network of roads to pharmaceutical hell.)

Atromid-S, the drug in question, was developed in England, where it had been tested for several years in the treatment of atherosclerosis. Diabetic patients suffering from associated atherosclerosis have been treated experimentally, both in England and the United States, with Atromid-S. In a number of persons who also had diabetic retinopathy retinal damage was checked, and according to some medical scientists has even been reversed.

Considerably more testing with many more patients will be necessary before any clear conclusions can be reached regarding the value of this drug in treating diabetic retinopathy, but the fact remains that for the first time there is promise of possible medical treatment.

Retinopathy of Hypertension

The retinopathy of high blood pressure is different in several respects from that of diabetes. In hypertensive retinopathy the arterioles — the smallest of arteries that bring blood into the capillaries — become constricted.

However, the damage done to the eyes is very similar. Small blood vessels supplying the retina become deformed, some burst, causing small hemorrhages, and cloudy exudates, like patches of cotton wool, are discharged into the eyes. The relationship between this retinopathy and the underlying high blood pressure is so close that physicians classify the seriousness of the hypertension by the amount of eye damage they can see through the ophthalmoscope. The retinopathy of hypertension causes blindness somewhat less frequently than that of diabetes, because high blood pressure severe enough to produce blindness can kill the patient before destroying his sight.

Ordinarily, the retinopathy of hypertension can be controlled by adequate treatment of the high blood pressure. However, hypertension can suddenly become uncontrollable, and fail to respond to any of the standard forms of treatment. When that happens there is a concommitant worsening of the retinopathy.

A team of medical researchers at Georgetown University,

headed by Dr. Frank Finnerty, has attempted recently to bring runaway hypertension under control by a process of sharp and repeated lowering of the arterial pressure, by means of a drug called *diazoxide*. Not only was the blood pressure brought back to a point where it could be controlled by ordinary treatment, Dr. Finnerty reported, but in most of his patients the signs of retinal damage were largely eliminated.

Other scientists, who have been testing Atromid-S in hypertension, report dramatic improvement of the associated retinopathies, just as occurred in diabetes. In an area where people once faced serious eye damage and possible blindness, the prospects have certainly taken an encouraging turn for the better.

Uveitis: The Inflamed Interior 15

Uveitis, which is considered one of the major common problems in ophthalmology, is actually a group of diseases, involving inflammation of the vitreous, retina, and the uveal tract.

The iris, the ciliary body, and the choroid together are called the uveal tract, because when seen apart from the rest of the eye they have a deep purple color, like the color of Concord grapes. (Therefore the name *uvea* – Latin for grapes.) Whenever any one of these parts of the eye becomes inflamed, the others are almost invariably affected.

Several years ago, a group of doctors in Syracuse, New York, found in a house-to-house survey that approximately two people in every thousand had uveitis. Another survey done in Rochester, Minnesota, in 1962 produced strikingly similar results. Otherwise there are no exact figures showing the incidence of uveitis, because as a noncontagious disease it is not reported to the U.S. Public Health Service. But on the basis of these two surveys, perhaps four hundred thousand people in the United States have uveitis.

The amount of blindness uveitis causes is not known, but Dr. A. Edward Maumenee, director of the Wilmer Ophthalmological Institute in Baltimore, has declared that it is responsible for an estimated 10 to 20 percent of all blindness.

Apart from its possibly serious consequences, what makes uveitis a major problem is the pattern of its occurrence. It most frequently strikes children under the age of thirteen, and adults between thirty and fifty, thus incapacitating its victims during two of the most important periods of their lives — when their learning patterns are being established in school, and during the years of their highest potential earning power.

Fortunately, the treatment of much uveitis has been aided by the new anti-inflammatory drugs, such as cortisone and other steroids.

Uveitis is considered a group of diseases because it includes at least six types of inflammation, with different causes, involving different parts of the uveal tract and requiring some variation in therapy.

One form, frequently seen in association with rheumatoid arthritis and other rheumatic diseases, is *acute nongranulomotous iridacyclitis*. This inflammation involves the iris and ciliary body, and unlike most other types of uveitis is usually self-limiting — that is, even if not treated, it runs its course in two or three weeks and then clears up, leaving very little damage to the eyeball.

Unfortunately, recurrence is frequent, and a number of these attacks may provoke cataract or secondary glaucoma.

A second type of uveitis has been traced to specific microbes that cause systemic diseases, such as tuberculosis, sarcoidosis, leprosy, syphilis, and others. People suffering from these diseases then develop the ocular inflammation as a consequence of the migration of the bacteria or viruses to the eye via the bloodstream.

A third type of uveitis, rare but particularly interesting because of its unusual cause, occurs mainly in children. This is produced by a parasite common to dogs, a roundworm called *Toxocara canis.* This worm is transmitted to children playing with infected puppies, eating dirt in which the eggs of the roundworm have been deposited.

One of the most thoroughly studied forms of uveitis, according to Dr. Maumenee, is caused by another parasite, *Toxoplasma gondi,* which is said to infect one out of every four people in the United States. Most often this parasite, which is frequently detected during routine examinations for something else, causes no trouble at all, but occasionally it will produce chills, fever, and inflammation of the lungs, heart, or brain. When it attacks the eyes, which it sometimes does in both children and adults, it produces an inflammation of the retina and choroid.

The fifth type of uveitis, occurring mainly in people between twenty and fifty, attacks both eyes, causing hemorrhages in the visual centers of the retina, and frequently results in blindness. Dr. Maumenee and his associates at the Wilmer Institute, studying this inflammation, have been unable to find any infecting organism in the affected eyes. Nonetheless, 94 percent of the persons with this ailment also have had a positive response to a skin test for a particular fungus – *Histoplasma capsulatum.* This microscopic mold is airborne and can be transmitted through contaminated dust, particularly in the countryside. While no direct cause-effect relationship has been established, the association appears more than coincidental.

Possibly the most unusual of all varieties of uveitis appear to be caused by autoimmunity, an abnormality in the process whereby people ordinarily fight off infections. In such cases, the process is turned against the person's own tissues, rather than against the invading organism. The disease-fighting mechanisms of the body cease to recognize the uvea as a normal part of the organism, and attack it as though it were a foreign substance. It is as though the body has become allergic to a part of itself and sets out to destroy it.

Autoimmunity is being investigated as a possible factor in a wide range of disease, from ulcerative colitis to rheumatoid arthritis.

There are a number of other forms of uveitis, caused by wounds, tumors, or ulcers, and some uveitis exists for which no specific cause has been found. One likely culprit is an untreated mature cataract. Once a cataract has ripened it usually begins to deteriorate, and may break up, releasing materials into the eye which might themselves cause uveitis, or possibly stimulate autoimmunization.

Because of its many possible causes and forms, uveitis presents the doctor with a difficult treatment problem.

First of all, he must identify the type of inflammation and determine the condition that lies at its root. He will probably examine the eye with an ophthalmoscope and a slit-lamp microscope which will enable him to study the tissues inside the eye.

He will perform blood tests, tests for possible infecting organisms, and skin tests for allergic reactions. Certainly a thorough physical examination will be necessary, and possibly additional examinations by specialists.

While a search is being made for the underlying cause of uveitis, the inflammation itself is not ignored. As we have noted,

View through ophthalmoscope of hemorrhagic lesion in the macular area of the retina of patient with uveitis.

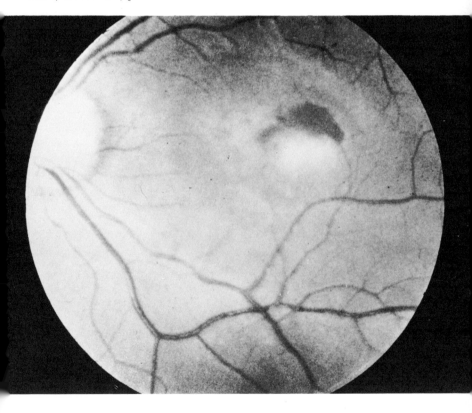

cortisone and the other drugs belonging to the cortical steroid group are especially effective in reducing inflammation. These drugs also may provide another advantage, in that they are often effective against autoimmunization. If a particular case of uveitis is caused by autoimmunity, the cortisone will serve a double purpose: to relieve the inflammation and strike at its cause.

There is no question but that uveitis can be very serious, but much of it can be successfully treated. As continuing research provides more knowledge as to its causes, the treatment is steadily improving.

Vitreous and the Optic Nerve 16

The vitreous body, which keeps the portion of the eye behind the lens filled out to its proper shape in much the same way as the air in a basketball keeps it inflated, is at birth a jellylike substance. With aging the jelly begins to lose its consistency, and gradually liquefies, sometimes becoming a factor in detachment of the retina. In the old, the vitreous has the appearance of a thickish liquid.

Since light must pass unimpeded and undistorted from the lens to the retina, the vitreous through which this light travels must be transparent. Any discoloration will cause some disturbance of vision, and any variations in the density of the vitreous can cause changes in light transmission and distort what we see. "Spots" before our eyes are actually bits of opaque material, known as *vitreous floaters,* floating within the vitreous and blocking some of the light rays. Hemorrhages, inflammation, or injuries to the eye may cause scraps of material, such as red blood cells or shreds of tissue, to enter the vitreous and cast shadows upon the retina.

Most damaging changes to the vitreous result from occurrences to other parts of the eye, ranging from infections to injuries, not only injecting such foreign matter as toxins and microorganisms into the vitreous, but often also speeding its liquefaction.

Wounds to the outer eye may penetrate to the vitreous and result in serious inflammations. Iron particles and some other metals that fly into the eye can be particularly dangerous, and should be removed as swiftly as possible.

Disorders of the Optic Nerve

The optic nerve, lying at the back of the eye, collects the light patterns formed on the retina and transmits them to the appropriate portion of the brain for evaluation and interpretation. Consisting of approximately five hundred thousand nerve fibers, the optic nerve passes from the back of the eye through the bony orbit for a distance of about an inch. Joining the nerve from the other eye, it sends its fibers back to the *visual cortex* at the rear of the brain.

All along this path, the optic nerve may be exposed to disturbances that will affect its function. Within the eye, the optic disk may become swollen. This condition, *papilledema,* may be caused in various ways, all of which produce an increase of fluid pressure within the skull.

Vision is not disturbed too much in the early stages of papilledema, but the blind spot gradually enlarges, and blindness may ensue unless the condition is treated. In treating papilledema, the physician will attempt to identify and alleviate the condition that causes the increase in fluid pressure. Once this is corrected, the swelling of the optic nerve usually subsides.

Another disease affecting the optic nerve is *papillitis,* or *optic neuritis*. It could result from some other primary inflammation such as sinusitis, meningitis, or an inflammatory disease of the brain itself, encephalitis. It could be the result of syphilis, multiple sclerosis, or some acute infective disease anywhere in the body. Finally, it might be caused by poisoning. Methyl alcohol, carbon tetrachloride, lead, and thallium can all produce optic neuritis.

The disease itself usually attacks only one eye, and the only symptom at the outset is a reduction of the field of vision. This may be minor or completely blinding. The maximum reduction in vision is usually reached within one or two days after the onset of the disease, at which point moving the affected eyeball may become painful.

While optic neuritis may take several months to run its course, early treatment of the optic inflammation with steroid drugs, as well as correction or alleviation of the underlying cause, will usually bring relatively full restoration of sight. It is also possible that, in some instances, the neuritis will clear up by itself — undergo a remission. But in the majority of cases, optic neuritis will result in partial blindness if it is untreated or if treatment is too long delayed.

There are a number of other disorders affecting the optic nerve along its course to the visual cortex of the brain. Generally, these are all due to other inflammatory conditions or diseases, problems in circulation, or toxic chemicals. A typical condition is *toxic amblyopia,* which produces a loss of visual acuity in both eyes and is most often caused by excessive smoking or alcoholic indulgence. Certain drugs can also cause this condition on occasion, as well as prolonged exposure to carbon monoxide, carbon tetrachloride, benzene, lead, and arsenic.

Since a number of the chemicals that can cause toxic amblyopia and optic neuritis are contained in cleaning fluids or paints — carbon tetrachloride, lead, and thallium, for instance — extreme care should be taken to avoid either physical contact or inhalation when using these substances. Many of us do not realize it, but eye damage and even blindness can result from using certain cleaning fluids and paints carelessly and without adequate ventilation.

Finally, there is a degenerative disorder, *optic atrophy,* that attacks the optic nerve and produces a progressive loss of vision. Its causes are not fully understood, but a number of conditions have been known to lead to this very serious disturbance, which usually results in blindness. Hereditary factors have been implicated, disorders of the blood circulation, toxic conditions, inflammations, and other situations that may interfere with the normal nutrition and chemistry of the optic nerve.

Because the damage resulting from optic atrophy cannot be reversed, it becomes all the more important for any unexplained reduction in vision to be diagnosed as quickly as possible so that prompt measures can be taken to discover the underlying cause and check its course.

Hazards to the Eye's 17 Exterior

The exterior of the eye is no less subject than the interior to inflammation, infection, and disease. Much of this is minor and heals without difficulty. Some can be serious, threatening sight. All can be worrisome.

When smoke, smog, or soap stings our eyes, what is irritated is not the eye itself but the protective membrane, the *conjunctiva*. Inflammation of this membrane, *conjunctivitis,* is one of the most frequent disturbances afflicting the eye. The inflammation can be produced by a variety of causes: chemical irritation, infections, allergic reactions, foreign substances, even disease in some other part of the body.

The first sign of conjunctivitis is usually a feeling of having some foreign body in the eye. The eye feels irritated, tears, becomes red. This may be followed by swelling and the appearance of a puslike substance in the eye. Pain, burning, or itching may occur, as well as a feeling of some sandy substance in the eye.

If there is no discharge of puslike fluid, the doctor will probably conclude that the conjunctivitis is due to an inflammatory condition, possibly treating it with one of the steroid drugs, such as cortisone. If pus is being discharged, chances are that an infection is involved. In that case the doctor tests to identify the infecting microbe and treats the infection as well as the inflammation, by adding an antimicrobial drug to the steroid.

He may also look to see if the portion of the conjunctiva that lines the eyelids appears pale or milky. If it is, the inflammation is probably the result of an allergic condition. Here, too, he would most likely use one of the steroid drugs.

Since some types of conjunctivitis, known as *pink eye,* are contagious, it is important to follow the doctor's instructions in order to prevent the spread of the disease to others.

Caused by a tiny organism that is neither a virus nor a bacterium but has some of the properties of both, *trachoma* is a chronic disease that attacks the conjunctiva and cornea. According to a 1965 statement of the World Health Organization, trachoma is the "greatest single cause of progressive loss of sight." Current estimates of the number of people suffering from this disease place the figure at more than 500,000,000.

The disease is spread through families by close contact. The infecting organism may also be carried by insects, such as gnats and flies, although doctors are still debating this. According to Dr.

P. Thygeson of the University of California in San Francisco, "Spread is encouraged by poverty and poor hygiene, particularly in desert areas of the world where lack of running water makes normal cleansing procedures impossible."

Until 1938 the medical approach had remained unchanged since the days of ancient Egypt, consisting of the use of cauterizing chemicals, such as copper salts, recommended in the Ebers Papyrus some thirty-six hundred years ago. In 1938, the sulfonamide drugs were introduced and found to be effective when taken by mouth. Since then a number of antibiotic drugs have also proved able to control the infection. Unfortunately, the treatment has to be prolonged and does not always work well. Furthermore, when the cured person returns to the same impoverished environment where he contracted trachoma, the chances are that he will be reinfected.

For this reason, Dr. Thygeson is convinced that it will be necessary to develop new methods of treating this disease before it can be eradicated. At the present time, he says, "trachoma is still a major problem in our southwestern Indian and Mexican populations, and sporadic cases are still being seen in the white population."

Fortunately, the days of this scourge may be drawing to a close, as the result of a breakthrough achieved by scientists in Peking, who solved the problem of growing the trachoma microbes in relatively pure cultures outside the human body. Dr. Albert B. Sabin, who reported the finding in October, 1966, calls this a major step toward the development of a vaccine.

Other Conjunctival Problems

Except for trachoma and conjunctivitis, the conjunctiva is only rarely attacked by serious illness. What ailments do occur are usually minor, overcome with little difficulty.

Occasionally, a small blood vessel under the conjunctiva may burst, causing a *subconjunctival hemorrhage*. Since the blood spreads rapidly under the smooth membrane, it presents a far more alarming appearance than ordinary bloodshot eyes in which the blood vessels are merely dilated. Usually the hemorrhage will clear up gradually by itself, more rapidly if cold compresses are applied over the closed eye for five minutes several times a day. But the bleeding might be caused by some serious condition that is not immediately apparent, and a doctor should be called upon for examination and treatment.

Scars due to infection or injury may develop and require surgical correction. Tumors and other growths, often easily visible, may occur. These are generally not serious, but should be examined by a physician and removed if necessary.

Swelling of the conjunctiva, or *edema,* may be the result of some problem in circulation, or it may be a remote expression of disease in the kidneys or some other part of the body. It is generally relieved by treatment of the underlying condition.

The Eyelid

The eye's protective outer shutter, the lid, also encounters a few problems. The most common of these is a swelling, or edema, frequently due to a sty, or *hordeolum.* The eyelid seems to thicken, becomes inflamed; a growth like a blister may form and there may be a discharge of pus. Altogether, it can cause considerable discomfort.

There are two types of sty: an external one, generally at the edge of the lid; and an internal one that involves the conjunctival membrane on the lid's inner surface. Both types can usually be treated effectively by the application of hot compresses, together with medication that combines steroid and antimicrobial drugs. If an eyelash follicle is the focal point of an external sty, the doctor may remove the lash, which is often very helpful in speeding recovery.

Swelling of the lid may also be due to an allergy. Usually such allergies are no great problem to the physician, who treats them with cold compresses and steroids.

The eyelids are subject to a vast number of other disturbances, which fortunately do not occur very frequently. These include such bacterial infections as *erysipelas,* to name one of the more serious, and viral infections, such as *herpes zoster ophthalmicus.*

Muscular problems that make the eyelids droop or difficult to open can also interfere with sight. Hereditary defects, nerve damage, or disease elsewhere in the body can be an underlying factor in this situation. Whatever the cause, treatment is generally possible, and surgery can usually correct the disturbances if other means fail.

The Cornea

The cornea, the tough, transparent outer portion of the eye through which light enters, comprises about one-sixth of the eye's forward covering. The remaining five-sixths, the sclera — the white of the eye — reaches backward to cover the portion of the eye inside the bony orbit. The cornea covers the colored portion of the eye and is separated from the sclera by a faint groove.

Since the cornea is the portion of the eye through which light must pass, any disturbances, however slight, can interfere with vision. Many things can happen to the cornea. Like most other body tissues, it can be affected by disease processes. It is subject to infections, inflammations, injuries, congenital abnormalities, degenerative conditions, and tumors.

Because of the direct importance of the cornea in the act of seeing, even the slightest disturbance should prompt a visit to an ophthalmologist.

Infections of the cornea once accounted for a considerable amount of damage. They produced ulcers, erosions, and opacities, frequently resulting in loss of the eye. Since the opening of the antibiotic era such infections are no longer as dangerous, provided they receive appropriate medical treatment. However, all corneal infection and inflammation, known under the general name of *keratitis,* is serious, because it can produce scarring over the area of the pupil, obstructing vision.

Dr. Arthur Gerard DeVoe, of Columbia University in New York, recently evaluated the present state of corneal disease thus: "Bacterial infections play a relatively minor role in present-day corneal disease. In the absence of neglect, most can readily be brought under control with the available medical agents."

Viral diseases and infections due to fungi do not respond to treatment as readily, Dr. DeVoe added. "Fungal infections of the cornea, like viral disease, have been increasing rapidly in the last few years and, since medications available for this condition are far from satisfactory, fungus keratitis remains one of our major problems."

Medical prevention of congenital deformities or of degenerative defects of the cornea is still not possible. A number of these can be corrected with eyeglasses or with surgery — particularly with corneal transplantation.

Injuries to the cornea are also increasing, according to Dr. De Voe. "We will have these with us as long as we have war, high-speed transportation, heavy machinery, and human carelessness," he declared.

Prompt attention to any injury, however slight, may make the difference between blindness and continued sight. The smallest foreign body in the eye, a speck of dust or ash, should be removed at once by a person trained in first aid, lest it cause inflammation and possible infection of the conjunctiva and sclera.

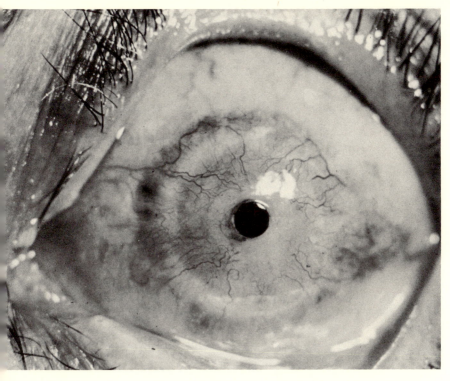
Eye with corneal transplant performed at Columbia University.

Damage to the cornea, whether from injury, infection, degenerative disease, or congenital abnormalities, results in defects in the shape of this "window," the formation of scar tissue, or a loss of transparency due to clouding or opacity. Each of these consequences will diminish vision, and in some cases obliterate it.

There are several ways of treating these effects of corneal damage. In some cases, contact lenses may correct the visual impediment, but they are not always helpful. Sometimes diseased corneal tissue can be removed by cauterization. For the most part, when serious permanent damage to vision seems likely, the situation may still be saved with a corneal transplant, from one of the eye banks that have been established in the United States for the express purpose of providing healthy corneas for transplantation. The eye banks receive their material from donors who leave their eyes to be donated after death, or from individuals whose eyes have to be removed for some condition that does not damage the cornea. The corneas from these eyes are preserved and stored until needed.

Unlike transplanted kidneys and other organs of the body, corneal transplants are not subject to attack and destruction by the body's immunity defenses against foreign substances. For this reason, the grafting of corneal tissue has been used successfully since early in the twentieth century.

The modern era of successful corneal transplantation dawned in 1924 with the work of V. P. Filatov in Russia, who gave this procedure an acknowledged place in eye surgery. His work was followed by that of Tudor Thomas in England in 1930, and Ramon Castroviejo in the United States in 1931.

Banks for Donated Eyes

It has been estimated that one blind child or adult out of every twenty-five could be helped by a corneal transplant from a donated eye. Donated eyes, moreover, also serve an important research purpose, making it possible to gain a better understanding of diseases that afflict the eyes, how to treat them, and, possibly, how to prevent them.

In order to make donated eyes available for these vital purposes, the first eye bank in the United States was established in 1944 by the Lions Club of Central Staten Island, New York. The idea spread, and in 1961 the Eye-Bank Association of America was founded by the American Academy of Ophthalmology and Otolaryngology. Today, with headquarters in Winston-Salem, North Carolina, the Eye-Bank Association has branches in practically every state in the nation.

Only adults can voluntarily donate their eyes. This is usually done by signing a regular form provided by the nearest Eye-Bank and having it witnessed by two disinterested adults. The original of this form is sent to the Eye-Bank, and a copy kept by the donor's next of kin.

In the event of the donor's death, the next of kin should notify the physician or hospital authorities of the donation immediately, since the eyes must be removed as soon as possible, preferably within one hour of and no later than four hours after death. Because of the need to remove the eyes promptly after death, before the process of deterioration begins, simply making a bequest in the will is useless. Too much time must necessarily pass before the provisions of a will are put into effect. If there is any objection on the part of the donor's immediate family, the eyes will not be taken.

Minors' eyes cannot usually be donated in advance, but permission to use the eyes may be given by the next of kin at the time of death.

More complete information can be obtained from the Eye-Bank Association of America, at 2041 Queen Street, Winston-Salem, North Carolina, 27103.

Preserved tissue for corneal transplant being removed from refrigerator by Mr. Capella, of the University of Florida, who developed much of the tissue preservation techniques.

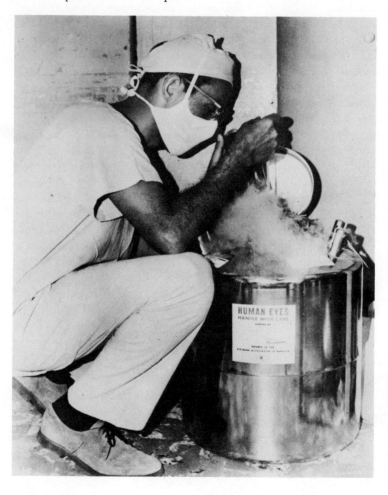

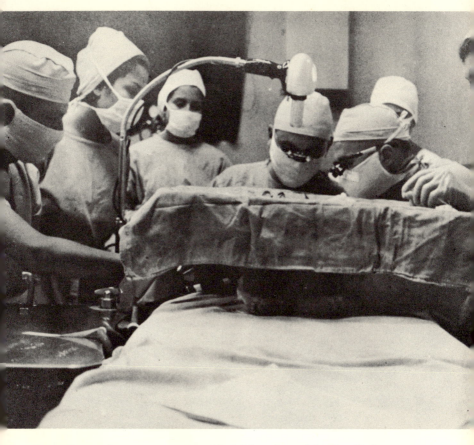

Corneal transplant on a two-year-old child performed by Dr. Herbert E. Kaufman at the University of Florida. Preserved graft on the blind child has remained clear and child now sees.

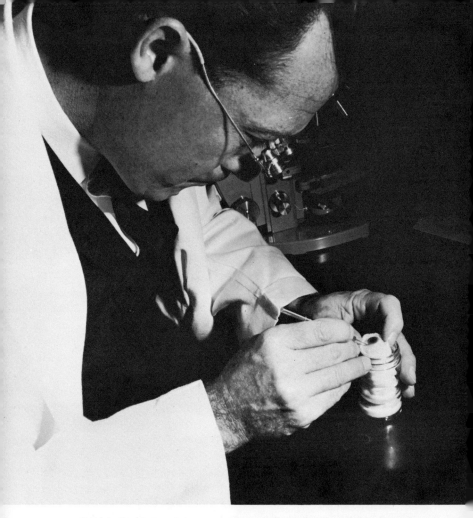

Dr. T. E. Moore, Jr., prepares to remove corneoscleral ring from preserved eye for possible transplant. University of California Medical Center, San Francisco.

In 1966, at a meeting sponsored by Research to Prevent Blindness, Inc., Dr. Herbert E. Kaufman of the University of Florida reported a new technique for keeping donated corneal tissue alive in a state of suspended animation. The corneas are placed in a mixture of dimethylsulfoxide, albumin and sucrose and then frozen at a precisely controlled rate to 190 degrees below zero centigrade. This technique, according to Dr. Kaufman, provides corneal material for transplant that remains clear and compares with freshly removed corneas.

When a transplantation operation is performed, the damaged portion of the cornea is removed and a matching section of donor cornea is sewn in to take its place.

Ordinarily, corneal transplantation is a successful procedure, with the new section of cornea remaining clear and useful. However, in a number of patients undergoing this operation, the grafts become opaque or abnormally crowded with blood vessels. In order to help these individuals, who would otherwise be blind, there has recently been a surge of interest in the possible use of artificial corneas made of some of the newer plastic materials. (See Chapter 26.)

The Sclera

The tough white sheath that encloses the globe of the eye appears more resistant to inflammation than the cornea. However, it is not totally immune.

Episcleritis, an inflammation of the outer portion of the sclera, can evoke discomfort or deep pain. Its cause is unknown and it is accompanied by nodules or patches, reddish-purple in color, usually located on the side of the eye nearest the temple.

Much more serious, potentially, is *scleritis,* an inflammation of the inner sclera, often occurring in association with rheumatoid arthritis. The pain is severe; there is tearing and considerable sensitivity to light. Dark purple nodules or patches appear on the sclera, sometimes even surrounding the cornea.

Untreated, scleritis may cause considerable damage to the sclera as well as other parts of the eye, resulting in impaired vision and even blindness.

Since both of these scleral inflammations are often difficult to distinguish from conjunctivitis, it is very important to see a physician or ophthalmologist as quickly as possible whenever any redness occurs. In scleritis, prompt diagnosis and treatment could be literally eye-saving.

In some people, as a result of severe infection or because of an abnormally elongated eyeball, the sclera may become thin, resulting in a condition known as *staphyloma*. When this occurs in the front portion of the sclera, it appears as a darkened area that bulges somewhat. Inside the orbit, staphyloma can only be seen through an ophthalmoscope.

The bulge seen in staphyloma is due to the pressure of the fluids inside the eyeball against a thin, weakened outer covering. The treatment, as in glaucoma, consists of reducing this pressure in order to prevent the thin section of sclera from being forced out even more, or even bursting.

Wounds to the sclera, when they occur in front of the eye, are clearly visible, because the darker interior layer of the eye, the choroid, can be seen through the injury. Whenever such a wound is detected, it should receive medical treatment at once.

Apart from these hazards and possible cysts and tumors, which occur only rarely, the sclera is relatively impervious, performing its protective and structural task of enclosing the eye effectively and with a minimum of trouble.

Tumors and Other Problems 18

Because they can usually be detected early, tumors involving the eye offer a better outlook for cure than tumors in other parts of the body.

Retinoblastoma, one of the most common cancers affecting the eyes of children, was nearly invariably fatal only a few years ago. Today it is almost 100 percent nonfatal, if it is recognized early and treated promptly. Prospects have also improved for *rhabdomyosarcoma,* the most common malignant tumor affecting the bony orbits of children. Dr. Algernon B. Reese of Columbia University says: "Such tumors . . . have a relatively good prognosis when prompt surgery is accepted."

In other types of cancer affecting the eye, such as *choroidal melanoma* and *orbital lymphoma,* the overall cure rate is approximately 50 percent. These figures, says Dr. Reese, highlight the importance of early diagnosis in the cure of all cancer.

Some of these tumors can be treated only surgically; others can be brought under control by the careful use of radiation, combined with anticancer chemicals. In using this combination therapy, the most modern approach to the treatment of retinoblastoma, the physician must achieve a delicate balance. Too much radiation may destroy the eye; too little may not destroy the tumor. Too small a dose of the cell-destroying chemicals would be ineffective; too large a dose might do serious damage to healthy parts of the body. So a balance is struck, with just enough of each form of treatment — radiation and chemotherapy — applied to eliminate the tumor without injuring the patient.

Benign tumors in various parts of the eye should also be treated promptly lest they do permanent damage. Some of these, of course, are readily apparent. Others can be seen only with the use of an ophthalmoscope. Even these will cause some disturbance — pain, a defect in vision, redness or hemorrhage, perhaps a protrusion of the eyeball if the tumor is located in the orbit. Any of these symptoms, or any other abnormality, should signal the need for a prompt visit to the doctor.

Lacrimal Disorders

The lacrimal apparatus that washes and lubricates the eyes provides important protection against irritation, inflammation, and infection. Occasionally, however, it may itself become a source of trouble.

Tears flow constantly through the eye. Leaving through the lacrimal ducts at the inside corner of the eye, they are brought to the lacrimal sac located alongside the nose. From the sac they are dispersed to the inside of the nose, where they evaporate. Inflammation of this sac, *dacryocystitis,* produces tearing, pain, and tenderness, plus redness and swelling of the area between the lower eyelid and the nose where the sac is located. There may also be a discharge of pus at the inner corner of the affected eye.

Most often this inflammation is caused by some obstruction of the tear ducts leading to the sac. In adults, such obstructions result from injuries to the nose, deviated septum, nasal inflammations, and other disturbances; in children, they are usually genetic in origin.

Antibiotic or antibacterial drugs, along with hot compresses over the affected area, will often be used by the ophthalmologist to treat dacryocystitis. If an abcess has formed, minor surgery may become necessary in the form of an incision and drainage.

If the inflammation is due to obstruction of the tear duct, this condition should also be treated. Lacrimal duct obstruction, called *dacryostenosis,* occurs most often in children. One of its signs is persistent tearing, generally from one eye. Ordinarily there is no difficulty in correcting this obstruction. Occasionally, when there is complete bony blockade of the duct, a new opening may have to be made surgically.

A drying up of tears, rather than an overflow, is very likely the result of some abnormality of the lacrimal gland where tears are produced, possibly damage to one of the nerves involved in its function.

Trouble in the Orbit

The protective bony socket in which the eye moves is subject to several hazards of its own. The bones of the orbit can be injured by blows or accidents, frequently resulting in infection of the orbit itself. Such an inflammation, called *orbital cellulitis,* may also be the result of the spread of infection from the teeth, the nasal sinuses, or other parts of the body.

Whenever possible the cause of the infection should be treated, as well as the orbital infection itself. Antibiotic or antibacterial drugs will probably be prescribed by the physician, along with bed rest, hot compresses to the affected area, and plenty of fluids. Unless it is corrected promptly, orbital cellulitis could very well have serious consequences, such as optic neuritis or an inflammation of the veins leading from the orbit and face.

Most orbital troubles produce protrusion of the eyeball, *exophthalmos*. This is often corrected when the underlying condition is cured. Occasionally, in severe exophthalmos, the doctor may find it necessary to perform surgery.

Because exophthalmos is invariably a clue that something is wrong with the eye or its environment, prompt medical attention should be sought as soon as it occurs. The protruding eyeball may well be the first sign of anything from a tumor to an inflammation, from a vitamin deficiency to a disorder of the thyroid gland. The doctor, knowing its significance, will probably use a variety of tests to pinpoint the precise cause. Once this has been done, it will be extremely important to follow his advice regarding treatment.

The Sensitive Eye 19

The function of pain is to warn of potential damage or danger. Through our evolutionary development, pain-sensitive nerve ends, or *receptors,* are distributed over various parts of our bodies in almost direct proportion to the importance of the involved parts. The greater the number of pain receptors in the area, the higher the sensitivity to pain. The ear lobe or the sole of the foot, for instance, have fewer receptors than the armpit or the groin; the eye, far more vulnerable than the other parts of the body surface, has a far higher concentration. A blow that would be painless to the sole of the foot would cause considerable pain in the groin, and agony on the eye.

The logic is simple. If the sole of the foot had more pain receptors, we would be unable to walk comfortably. If the eye had fewer pain receptors, we would not be aware of irritations, inflammations, and other potentially dangerous situations that could seriously damage or destroy it.

The eye's extreme sensitivity does more than merely protect that organ; it also alerts us to danger to other parts of the body. Often, because of the eyes' greater sensitivity, our first awareness of something wrong in another part of the body comes to us through the eyes. Certain disease conditions often produce swelling, inflammations, visual defects, and other changes.

Clues to a great many diseases can be seen in the eyes. Anemia and leukemia cause changes in the blood vessels of the retina, as well as a pallor in the blood vessels on the conjunctiva of the eyelid. Tumors, infections, and diseases affecting the brain will often produce swelling of the optic nerve. The first signs of multiple sclerosis, the crippling disease that affects the nervous system, are often a fleeting paralysis of the orbital muscles, double vision, dimness of vision, or the appearance of blind spots.

Glandular disturbance of various sorts can also be seen through changes in the eyes, as can metabolic diseases involving abnormalities in the body's chemistry.

Changes in the blood vessels of the retina are often very early signs of diabetes. The degree of hypertension is often classified on the basis of abnormal changes in the retina. Kidney disease may cause swelling of the eyelids and the conjunctiva, as well as disturbances of the retina. Abnormal functioning of the thyroid gland might be betrayed by protruding eyeballs.

An inadequate diet producing nutritional deficiencies often affects the eyes. An association between a vitamin deficiency and night blindness is fairly common, and the lack of other vitamins may be involved in ocular hemorrhages, optic neuritis, and other abnormal conditions.

Linked with the retinopathies associated with diabetes and hypertension are atherosclerosis, or hardening of the arteries, and what is generally known as occlusive vascular disease — disturbances due to interference with the circulation. These circulatory ailments may affect the eyes in two ways — by producing damage to the blood vessels of the retina, causing hemorrhages and other injuries that could interfere with sight; and by reducing the flow of blood to the eye, depriving it of the oxygen and nutrients it needs in order to function properly. Occasionally atherosclerosis chokes off the central retinal artery, one of the main arteries feeding the eye, which can produce serious damage to vision.

The eye's accessibility augments its importance as a key to the detection of disease in other parts of the body. Not only are eye pain and other abnormalities readily experienced, but the particular changes involved can be easily seen. Even those that occur deep within the eye, at the retina or the cup of the optic nerve, can be examined with an ophthalmoscope or one of the other modern instruments that permit close study of the eye's interior and its function. With the aid of special motion picture equipment and a fluorescent dye injected into the circulating blood, it has even become possible to photograph the distinctive abnormalities of the tiny blood vessels that occur in diabetic, hypertensive, atherosclerotic, and other retinopathies. Similar blood vessel abnormalities occur in other parts of the body with these diseases — in the kidneys and brain, for instance. There they would go undetected without surgery to reveal them, but in the eye they are immediately visible.

Any complete physical examination by a physician usually involves examination of the eyes. If anything suspicious shows up, he will often use the ophthalmoscope for a fuller examination of the *optic fundus* — the rear of the eye where the retina lies. Examinations of the optic fundus are a regular part of the management of high blood pressure. By seeing whether or not improvement occurs in the blood vessels of the retina, the physician is able to judge whether or not the treatment he is prescribing is effective. He may also be able to predict the outcome of the disease by studying the retina.

German Measles

One of the most important diseases that produce secondary damage to the eyes is *German measles (rubella)*. The infants, who are the victims, do not directly contract the rubella; instead, it is the mother who has the disease during pregnancy.

The fact that severe congenital abnormalities occurred in the newborn infants of mothers who had suffered attacks of this viral disease during pregnancy was first recognized in 1941 by the Australian ophthalmologist, Sir Norman McAlister Gregg of the Royal Alexandra Hospital for Children in Sydney. That year, following an epidemic of rubella, Dr. Gregg noticed that there was a sudden and unexpected increase in the number of infants with congenital cataracts. This puzzled him, so he began an investigation, closely questioning the mothers of the affected infants. Of seventy-eight mothers, sixty-eight were able to remember having the viral infection during the first three months of the pregnancy, when the fetus was actually being formed.

Cataracts were not the only defects found in these infants. Dr. Gregg, who was later knighted for his findings, also observed that there was a higher than normal incidence of congenital heart defects, as well as infant mortality, associated with the maternal rubella. These findings were later confirmed by a number of other scientists.

Because the implications were so important, an intensive investigation was undertaken when there was a widespread rubella epidemic in the United States during the first half of 1964. Scientists found that the rubella virus often crossed the barrier of the placenta and infected the fetus with a chronic form of the disease that remained with the infant even after birth. Many of these newborn infants were also carriers of the disease, spreading the infection to those who came in contact with them.

At birth, the infected infants were of low weight, had enlarged livers and spleens, and a blood-clotting defect which made them bleed easily. In addition, cardiovascular abnormalities were observed, plus hearing defects, mental retardation, and a number of ocular abnormalities.

Apart from the cataracts, other features of the rubella syndrome in the eyes included abnormally small eyeballs (*microphthalmos*), glaucoma, defective irises and retinas, and a significant decrease in vision.

Recent studies at the University of California in Los Angeles have shown that while the ocular defects of such infants can be treated, the results generally leave a good deal to be desired. The most reasonable way of dealing with these defects is by preventing rubella in the mother during pregnancy. Attempts to use gamma globulin as a means of preventing the disease in pregnant women who have been exposed to the virus have so far shown doubtful results at best. "In fact," says Dr. Bradley R. Straatsma of UCLA, "it may even be detrimental in that it may mask the clinical manifestations of the disease and thus obscure its diagnosis, while not actually preventing the virus infection."

Recently, a vaccine against German measles has reportedly been developed. If successful, this might bring us a long step closer to the elimination of rubella-instigated blindness in children.

Inflammations and Autoimmunization

Rheumatoid arthritis and gout, although primarily diseases that affect the joints, also seem to be associated with a number of inflammatory conditions in the eye. This has caused scientists to wonder whether both inflammations — of the joint and of the eye — are due to the same cause, or whether the person subject to rheumatic disease or gout has a similar predisposition to inflammations of the eye.

Before these questions can be answered, much more will have to be learned about the autoimmunization process. Many scientists believe that a number of rheumatic and other inflammatory conditions are the direct result of the body's own disease-fighting apparatus turning on and attacking normal body tissue. This attack on one's own self is, in turn, due to a breakdown in identification signals, an inability to distinguish body cells from invading cells.

Some doctors consider it interesting and possibly significant that the drugs such as cortisone, which are effective in reducing inflammation, also have a depressing effect on the body's immune reaction. They suggest that these two effects may be related. If this is shown to be so, it could provide additional evidence of a link between autoimmunization and inflammatory disease.

Allergy and the Eyes

Anyone who suffers from hay fever knows that allergies affect the eyes. The range of various allergic effects upon our eyes is much greater than many people imagine, encompassing far more than sensitivities to pollen, animal hair, and dust. Drugs, cosmetics, heat, sunlight, and other factors normally found in our environment, even bacteria and other microorganisms, can all affect our eyes, causing swollen eyelids, inflammations of the conjunctiva or cornea, redness and tearing.

Allergies are often called *hypersensitivity reactions*. The body is exposed to a substance, such as a particular pollen, and becomes sensitive to it, just as though the pollen were an invading microbe. The next time the pollen is introduced, the body produces antibodies to attack it. Unfortunately, in an allergy state, this is not an ordinary reaction but an overreaction. Dr. G. Richard O'Connor, of the University of California San Francisco Medical Center, calls hypersensitivity "an exuberant reaction on the part of an animal host to invasion by a foreign element in his external environment."

Because of this overreaction, not only is the invading element or antigen attacked by the antibodies, but other parts of the body — innocent bystanders such as skin, eye, or nasal mucosa — are also involved. These innocent tissues are attacked, not by the antibodies as would be the case in an autoimmunization reaction, but by complex substances formed by antigen-antibody combinations.

Sympathetic ophthalmia, one of the most serious of the hypersensitivity reactions affecting the eye, is considered the classic form of this type of disease. It is a direct, destructive reaction affecting an otherwise healthy eye as the result of hypersensitivity induced by inflammation in the other eye.

Vernal conjunctivitis, a hypersensitivity that is apparently triggered by hot weather, is a childhood disease that recurs every spring for a period of from five to seven years, and eventually heals without complications. Because it is self-limiting, physicians tend to treat only the symptoms as they appear, and avoid using some of the potent drugs that might produce unwanted side effects.

Food allergies that produce hives may also involve the eyes, sometimes causing dramatic swelling of one or both eyelids. While this can be very alarming, the condition usually responds well to treatment with antihistaminic drugs. However, the best treatment is preventive — identifying the allergenic food, and avoiding it.

Contact blepharoconjunctivitis is another type of allergy that may cause inflammation of the conjunctiva and swelling of the lids, because of sensitivity to poison ivy, certain drugs, cosmetics, and other substances that primarily affect the skin through direct contact. If the doctor can identify the offending substance that causes the allergic response, this condition can be prevented. Sometimes, however, not even the most careful detective work can isolate the guilty allergen. In such cases, steroid therapy has been found very useful.

In treating contact blepharoconjunctivitis, the doctor will first make sure that the cause is not really *infectious eczematoid dermatitis* of the lids. This is a staphylococcus infection, although it resembles the more common contact allergy, and clears up very rapidly when the offending microbes are eliminated with antibiotic or antimicrobial drugs.

Whatever the particular type of allergy involved, prompt medical attention will usually alleviate it, hold off serious damage, and possibly prevent another occurrence.

3

PROTECTING YOUR SIGHT

Accidents and First Aid 20

An estimated 5 percent of all blindness in the United States is the result of injury. A much higher percentage of people suffer partial loss of vision, as well as considerable pain and anxiety, because of eye injuries. And most such injuries are the bitter fruit of accident, ignorance, or plain carelessness.

Contrary to the commonly held belief that infants are most subject to eye injury, the greatest risk of all seems to come during the junior high school years, probably the period of our greatest activity. The hazards are multiplied because that is also the time of the most dedicated devil-may-care attitude toward safety. Infants, in fact, although relatively helpless to protect themselves, are only minimally exposed to danger.

Adults, of course, have their share of eye injuries — a wood splinter lodged in the eye in the home workshop; a splash of ammonia in the eye while cleaning house; a branch slashing the eye in underbrush. The possibilities are endless, at work, at play, in the home.

The first rule of eye safety is: *Do not rub*. When hurt, most people almost reflexively press or rub the injured part. Where the eye is concerned, this could be ruinous. If there is a foreign object in the eye, rubbing may only lodge it more firmly, perhaps causing permanent damage. The same is true if acid or other corrosive material has entered the eye, or with other types of injury.

Another very important rule for eye safety is that no injured eye should be treated by anyone, no matter how closely related, how friendly, how gentle, or how trusted, who does not have medical training. Nor should any medication be used in an injured eye unless prescribed by a physician.

It used to be a fairly common practice to ask the neighborhood druggist to remove specks and other foreign bodies from our eyes, or to provide other first aid. The druggists, often accommodating, knowledgeable men, usually provided what first aid they could. Frequently this sufficed, but sometimes serious damage to the eye developed because first aid was simply not enough. While the druggist is a trained and highly skilled pharmacist, he generally has no training as a doctor or ophthalmologist.

When a foreign body enters the eye, the best thing to do is allow your tears to wash it out, if possible. Meanwhile, seek the prompt help of a nurse or someone specially trained in first aid. If the tears do not clear away the speck, and no trained person is immediately available, then, making sure your hands are clean, cover your closed eye loosely with a gauze dressing and go at once to a doctor or a nearby hospital or clinic.

Do not try to remove the foreign object with the corner of a handkerchief or cotton wool on a toothpick. Admittedly, this might frequently do the job, but too often it has caused infection and permanent damage to the cornea. Every foreign body carries bacteria. These can find a ready breeding place in the conjunctiva, particularly if that membrane has been irritated. Only a doctor is properly qualified to administer the appropriate antibacterial or antibiotic drug.

If the foreign body is not a mere speck on the surface, but has actually penetrated the eye, do not wait for tears or first aid to do the job, but cover the eye and go at once to the doctor.

Similarly, if the eye has been cut or scratched in any way whatsoever, do not attempt any first aid. Do not apply medication — do not even try to wash or clean the injured eye. Cover the eye loosely with a light gauze bandage and call an ophthalmologist or your physician at once.

Blows

Almost everyone has "walked into a door," fallen, or been struck in or near the eye with bats, balls, fists, rocks, or other missiles. A blow on the uncovered eye itself makes an immediate trip to the doctor imperative. If the eye was closed, however, and there is no apparent damage other than a possible black eye, first aid can be helpful.

Try applying cold compresses, keeping them on the struck area for about fifteen minutes. If pain, blurred vision or any consequent visual abnormality does not clear up within the first fifteen minutes following the accident, go to your doctor at once. Continued severe pain or blurriness may mean serious damage to the eye, or even to the bony orbit.

If the effects do clear up promptly and a trip to the doctor does not seem necessary, continue the cold compresses every hour, for at least five hours. This treatment may prevent the black eye from developing. If it does not, the application of raw steak or other cuts of meat will have absolutely no effect other than to help enrich the butcher. It may be helpful, though, to apply hot compresses, on the same schedule, starting the day after the accident. This should be of aid in clearing up the hemorrhages that produce black eyes.

In order to increase the odds in your favor, both to avoid the likelihood of serious damage from a blow and to prevent a black eye, the best thing to do is go to the doctor as soon as possible. By injecting the enzyme *hyaluronidase* in combination with pain-killing *procaine,* he can prevent or quickly clear up any possible black eye, and he will also be able to examine the eye and the orbit for any possible hidden damage.

Burns

Many things can burn the eyes — flames, sparks from cigarettes or matches, glowing ashes, intense heat from a furnace or electric arc, acids, alkalis, and other corrosive chemicals. Certain substances not ordinarily considered to be dangerous chemicals can produce serious burn injuries in the eye. Flakes of wall plaster, for instance, can cause progressive damage because they contain corrosive alkali. So, too, can a number of ordinary household cleansers.

If a spark, ash, chemical or other corrosive substance burns the eye, it is imperative that the eye be flooded immediately with cool or lukewarm running water for approximately fifteen minutes. If possible, hold the head under a faucet and allow the water to run over the open eye. If there is no faucet available, pour the water from a pot, a cup or whatever container is available, making sure that it is clean and that the water is clear. Do not use an eye cup or anything of that nature — a constant flow of water is absolutely essential.

Meanwhile, a doctor should be called immediately — without any delay whatsoever. Burns to the eye can be extremely damaging unless dealt with promptly and competently.

Fatigue

Ordinarily, eye fatigue is not fatigue of the eye at all, but a reflection of strain involving the various muscles that move and accommodate the eye. There are many reasons for this. Bad posture while using the eyes can cause muscle strain, as can improper lighting or fixed concentration of the eyes on a particular object.

The burning sensation often associated with eye fatigue might also be due to smog, smoke, or some other form of atmosphere contamination. It could also be a sign of inflammation or injury.

If the fatigue or burning sensation is not due to some unusual or dangerous circumstance, resting the eyes should be enough to provide relief. Look at something green, or close the eyes and apply cool compresses. Eyedrops or an eye rinse recommended by the doctor for just such an occasion may ease the eyes.

The best help for tired eyes, however, is prevention. When reading or working make sure that your posture is good and the lighting adequate, and allow your eyes to wander — do not keep them fixed too long on any single object. Try to avoid air that is polluted with too much dust, smoke, smog, and other contaminants. And of course if the condition persists, or is accompanied by changes in vision, pain, or inflammation, visit your physician.

21 Defending Your Eyes

Nature provided man's eyes with lids, lashes, and a tough outer skin and set them into a bony socket, in order to give them as much protection as possible without diminishing their function. But nature could not anticipate the modern hazards man was to create for himself, and natural selection has not yet weeded out those humans who are constitutionally unable to cope with such man-made perils as industrial accidents, smog, wars, automobile smashups, plane crashes, fireworks, flying glass, golfballs, baseballs, rifle backfires, and an infinity of other potentially killing or crippling embellishments of civilization. Until we and our eyes evolve some sort of protective armor plate against such threats, if we ever do, our sole protection is intelligent care and caution.

Most of the accidents that produce eye damage and blindness are avoidable; most of the illness that might end in blindness or permanent loss of vision can, if detected and treated early enough, be checked before any serious harm is done.

One of the first and most obvious rules of eye protection is to have regular examinations, performed by an opthalmologist, every two years. Furthermore, should the eyes give any trouble at all, become painful, inflamed, or abnormal in any way, they should be cared for at once.

Pain or inflammation are obvious signs of possible trouble, and chances are that you will notice them as soon as they occur. But a number of other danger signals develop so gradually that the ordinary person is not as conscious of them as he would be of pain, and many people tend to ignore them until serious damage has already been done.

The most important sign of a developing cataract is a gradual decrease of vision in the affected eye. Ordinarily this may be difficult to detect, since the good eye will tend to mask the fact that the other eye is not seeing well. It is wise to test the acuity of each eye separately from time to time.

Developing cataracts can be detected in strange ways. A professional photographer one day noticed that his camera did not seem to focus sharply. At first he thought the camera's lenses or finder might be fogged, so he cleaned them carefully and tried again. The image was still somewhat blurred. The next possibility that suggested itself was that the finder was somehow out of alignment. But before he tested this, he glanced through the finder with the other eye — and the image was sharp and clear. He tried the first eye again — blurred. The following day he was examined by his ophthalmologist, who discovered a cataract developing in the lens of the left eye.

Early diagnosis of cataracts will not necessarily have any

effect upon the outcome, since there is no medical or surgical treatment that can slow, stop, or reverse the process whereby the lens becomes opaque. On the other hand, the development of the cataract may slow, speed up, or stop entirely by itself. The reasons for this are not known but they must certainly involve some changes in the metabolic processes associated with cataract formation. One thing must be emphasized: Even if the cataract stops its progress, the damage already done to the lens will remain.

Early detection may not be particularly important as far as cataracts are concerned, but it can be sight-saving in the case of glaucoma and almost all the other disorders that affect the eyes. For this reason we must be alert for the subtler clues, those that do not force themselves upon our attention as do pain or inflammation.

> Among these signs are:
> The need to change eyeglass prescriptions frequently.
> Gradual loss of side vision.
> The appearance of rings, halos, or colored rays around lights.
> Blurred or foggy vision.
> An increased sensitivity to light.
> Difficulty in adjusting the eyes to a darkened room.
> Excessive tearing, or its opposite, a dryness of the eyes.
> Noticeable and prolonged eye blinking.
> Protrusion of the eyeballs.
> Uncontrolled rhythmic movements of the eyes.

As soon as any of the above signs are noticed, as well as any of the more obvious trouble warnings such as pain, inflammation, redness of the eyes, and so on, you should arrange a prompt visit to the ophthalmologist or family doctor.

DEFENDING YOUR EYES

Adults and adolescents have no trouble spotting any of these clues, once they are alert to them, but parents must be on the lookout for such signs in their children. Chapter 22 will take up the protection of young eyes.

Preventing most accidents requires only some imagination, intelligence, and a normal amount of caution. In trekking through heavy brush, you should be alert to the possibility of a branch snapping back into your face. In working with power tools, you should remember that wood or metal chips might fly and present some hazard to your eyes. In painting a ceiling, you need little imagination to know that paint is likely to drip down, perhaps into your eyes.

In every case where possible trouble is anticipated, defensive measures should be taken — wearing protective glasses or safety goggles, using transparent shields, or, in the case of painting a ceiling, using a dripproof roller as well as glasses or an eyeshade, just in case.

Taking that extra precaution to protect the eyes is an act of intelligent self-preservation. Undoubtedly there are some who feel that wearing safety goggles is somehow "chicken," like using a seatbelt in an automobile, or wearing a helmet on a motorcycle or to do a construction job. Such attitudes occur at all ages, and can sometimes prove tragic.

An important protective measure, particularly when doing hazardous work, is the wearing of goggles made of shatterproof glass. Some eye specialists even suggest that ordinary corrective eyeglasses be made of safety glass, to provide additional protection. Experimental safety lenses are now being made of plastic. These are lighter in weight, stronger, and more transparent than those made of glass, but they tend to scratch more easily. On the other hand, safety lenses made of glass tend to be heavier and somewhat thicker than regular glass lenses.

The Hazardous Sun

The sun, the source of life in our solar system, also provides a number of disguised and overt hazards to our eyes and skin. The American Medical Association's Council on Dermatology has for years published thoroughly documented warnings about the dangers of exposure to the sun's ultraviolet radiation. In addition to being a cause of skin cancer, these rays can permanently damage the retinas of the eyes. They can also instigate the process that will lead to cataract formation. In fact, some scientists believe that many cataracts in the elderly may simply be the result of the accumulated damage done over the years by sunlight and other factors.

Since we live, work, and play in the sun, it is important that we avoid its hazards while using its advantages. Never, under any circumstances, should anyone look directly into the sun, not even with the darkest sunglasses. Not only is the ultraviolet dangerous, but also the infrared and other solar radiation can cause permanent injury and lead to blindness.

Many pleasurable activities take place in strong sunlight — swimming, boating, golfing, gardening, picnicking, skiing, and driving. To protect our eyes, we should wear optically ground sunglasses, in winter as well as summer, especially if there is snow on the ground. For any activities that expose us to the full light of the sun, either directly or by reflection from snow, sand, water, concrete, or similarly reflective surfaces, the sunglasses should be dense enough to transmit only 20 to 30 percent of the sun's visible light, and to absorb some of the infrared and ultraviolet radiation as well. The color of sunglasses is not significant.

Finally, people who lie out in the sunlight for long periods to obtain a tan should keep their eyes closed, and wear protective pads of cotton over their closed eyelids.

Regardless of the dangers of sunlight, without light we would have no sight, and the best way to help the eyes do their job is to provide them with the most effective kind of lighting.

Recently, high-intensity lamps have come into a sort of vogue, supposedly as a means of helping support better vision. But on the contrary, these lights may actually do damage if used alone. The most effective and least damaging lighting should be neither too dim nor too bright, and it should not provide sharp contrast, as does a spotlight in an otherwise dark room. The light should provide enough illumination to see by comfortably, with no glare and no deep shadows.

Whether this light is provided by a fluorescent fixture, an incandescent lamp, or some other type of light source is not particularly significant. What is important is that the light source be sufficiently bright to illuminate all of the details so they can be seen clearly, without difficulty or strain.

The best light to use is bluish-white, one that simulates the color of daylight. Should you use a high-intensity lamp or some other form of supplementary lighting on work or reading matter, there should also be a soft light cast evenly over the entire working area. Actually, the whole room should have an evenly diffused light, one without glare that produces a minimum of shadows and harsh reflections. Some shielded type of overhead lighting is frequently best for this purpose, since it does not send its rays directly into the eyes.

In addition to the overall even room light, the work light or reading light being used should be so placed and shielded that you do not find yourself looking directly at the bulb. The old concept that the light should come over the right shoulder ought to be laid to rest. For reading purposes it makes no difference whether the light comes over the right or left shoulder, as long as you can read comfortably by it. But when doing any work — writing, sewing, carpentry — it is best to have light come over the left shoulder of a right-handed person, and the right shoulder of a left-handed person, to reduce the possibility of shadows being cast on the work.

Reading in bed is in no way harmful or injurious, as long as the light is suitable and the reader is in a comfortable position that does not produce muscular strain, especially on the neck and shoulders.

Proper diet, exercise, adequate rest, the maintenance of proper weight are as important to the health of the eyes as to the rest of our bodies. Early detection and treatment of atherosclerosis, high blood pressure, heart and circulatory disturbances, as well as most other systemic diseases and infections will have a protective effect upon the eyes. Even with the eyes in relatively "perfect" shape, you should have an ophthalmologic examination every two years. Not only will such regular examinations help protect your eyes, but they might also provide early clues to disease in other parts of the body. After the age of forty a complete eye examination annually is a virtually essential protective measure.

These precautions are a small price to pay for the well-being of your sight.

Protecting Children's Eyes 22

Dr. John W. Ferree, executive director of the National Society for the Prevention of Blindness, Inc., tells a story of a first-grade pupil who had her eyes examined as part of the school program. Wearing the prescribed glasses for the first time, she watched television with her mother. "Why, Mommy," she exclaimed delightedly upon looking at the screen, "those are people!"

A young child has no way of knowing whether his vision is good or bad. Since undetected vision defects can produce permanent damage, and since the child is unable to recognize these defects, adults are responsible for the care and protection of his eyesight.

The best time to start protecting a child's eyes is in his infancy. Before he is one year old he should be immunized against such contagious diseases as measles, smallpox, and diphtheria, all of which can damage the eyes. Measles is now known to be a far more serious cause of eye damage than had previously been suspected.

The parent must also realize that the average pediatrician's study frequently neglects the infant's eyesight. Of course this is not always the case; many pediatricians do check the eyes as well. But when a mother is told that her child is in excellent health, she should ask specifically if this clean bill includes the eyes.

The first test by an ophthalmologist should take place no later than age four. Crossed eyes or some other obvious defect should be attended to as soon as it is noticed. Dr. Gunter K. von Noorden of Johns Hopkins University Medical School is particularly emphatic about this. "The old erroneous notion that strabismus or crossed eye usually outgrows itself or does not need to be corrected until school age must be eliminated," he insists. "Treatment for eye-muscle imbalance and thus for its consequence, the amblyopic eye, is possible in any child after the age of six months."

Since amblyopia may also occur in seemingly normal eyes, this defect is often not noticed until the first examination upon entering school. By then it is usually too late to prevent permanent damage. This is particularly ironic because up until the age of four amblyopia can be cured in virtually every instance. Failure to make a routine eye examination a standard part of every child's health program risks unnecessary single-eye blindness. In a recent Air Force eye examination, Dr. Ferree points out, more than two hundred of the five thousand men examined were found to be suffering from significant loss of sight in one eye as a result of amblyopia.

A parent can give the preschool child a number of tests to prepare him for his first ophthalmologic examination. One of the

PROTECTING CHILDREN'S EYES

most effective, suggested by the Children's Eye Clinic at Presbyterian Hospital in New York, is a modification of the Snellen E test, a standard method used to measure the visual acuity of children.

In black crayon on a white card draw a large capital E, measuring about six inches in every direction. Hold the card up, with the child standing ten feet away, and have him cover each eye separately and tell you which way the "legs of the table" are pointing. Have him point the direction as you change the position of the E, repeating the test at least seven times.

Neither this test nor any other a parent may give should be considered as conclusive one way or the other, although it is good preparation and may give a preliminary indication of trouble. Only an ophthalmologist is qualified to judge the health of a child's eyes, or anyone else's.

Almost every state in the union has compulsory dental examinations for children starting school, but fewer than half have mandatory eye examinations. Furthermore, tests that are adequate to detect trouble in adults are often less effective in children. A child might have two good eyes and still have a defect in vision. Each eye, checked separately, may appear perfectly normal — actually be perfectly normal — yet the child may be seeing double, or his eyes may be seeing images of different sizes. Some children have mirror vision; they see certain objects backward.

These and similar defects are often faults in the way the nervous system and brain interpret, rather than in the eyes themselves. Such problems can be corrected, of course, but first they have to be detected. And this cannot be done if the child is given a cursory eyechart test for each eye separately. All that the chart test determines is whether or not the child has 20/20 vision in each eye. It does not show whether or not he can see comfortably at reading distance. It cannot spot double vision, or any of the other defects that arise from the brain's misinterpretation of what the child sees.

Assembly-line chart tests for schoolchildren are simply not enough. The eyes must not only be examined separately but together to determine how well they function as a team. Furthermore the examinations must be repeated at regular intervals, since the eyes of children are subject to considerable change during the period of rapid growth.

It is senselessly damaging and tragic for a child to be labeled "dull," "backward," or "stupid" because of an undetected defect in vision. Such an error can often lead to personality disturbances that mar a child's entire life.

One seven-year-old boy's chart test showed him to have 20/20 vision, but despite his apparently normal sight he had a number of problems. He had great difficulty learning to read and write, he seemed unable to concentrate, he was awkward at games, he couldn't learn to catch or throw a ball properly. He was physically clumsy, not at all well coordinated.

The boy's classmates derided and made fun of him, and the teacher, after a period of scolding him for slowness and inattention, accepted him as a cross she had to bear and ignored him. The boy reacted by withdrawing, refusing to play, even refusing to speak to others.

The child's mother, rejecting the idea that her son was "stupid," sought desperately for some answer. The family doctor, finding nothing wrong with him physically, suggested a thorough eye examination.

It did not take the ophthalmologist long to spot the trouble. The boy was suffering from a form of *diplopia* — double vision. It was this, rather than stupidity, that made it difficult for him to read and write, to concentrate on his lessons, to catch and throw a ball accurately, to coordinate.

Once the trouble was detected, the correction was relatively easy. But the psychological damage done to this child, his sense of strangeness and inferiority, will probably be far more difficult to heal.

Children with perfectly good vision sometimes develop eye defects as they grow older, for a number of possible reasons: Illness, injury, metabolic disturbances, glandular changes, hereditary abnormalities that take time to manifest themselves. Whatever the reason, the most immediate result of the change in vision will be a decline in scholastic performance.

Just as every "backward" child should have a complete eye examination, so should a child who suffers an unexplained drop in learning ability. Sudden bad marks may have nothing at all to do with the child's intelligence, but be a clue to existing or developing eye trouble.

Often the trouble can be remedied with corrective glasses, or a change in the child's prescription. Sometimes more complex measures are necessary. But whatever the problem, chances are that it can be corrected if it is discovered promptly.

It is not safe to assume that just because a child's vision has been rated as perfect, it will remain so. The child's eyes grow along with the child. Changes are constantly taking place; what is "perfect" vision one year may be imperfect the next year, or even in a few months.

Occasionally, of course, it is virtually impossible for parents to notice the signs of a defect, but these situations are rare. Most of the time the signs are plain enough, and are overlooked only because of ignorance or inattention. Periodic examinations are extremely important, and parents should also be alert for the following possible clues to developing trouble:

Does the child
rub his eyes excessively?
frequently stumble over small objects?

YOUR SIGHT: FOLKLORE, FACT AND COMMON SENSE

often squint or frown?

seem to be trying to brush something away from in front of his eyes?

squint when looking at distant objects?

hold objects close to his eyes to look at them?

hold his head far forward, or tilt his head, or close one eye when looking at something?

seem overly sensitive to light or have trouble seeing when going from a dark room to a light room, or vice versa?

have inflamed or red eyes, or inflamed eyelids?

have trouble catching a ball or other objects tossed to him?

seem to be doing badly in school, or have difficulty reading?

fumble small objects he is handling?

Should any of these twelve signs appear, do not wait until the child's next examination to mention it; arrange a prompt appointment with the ophthalmologist. The chances are that nothing serious is involved; but delay could be dangerous.

About four out of every ten eye injuries to children are the result of direct blows from fists, balls, or the like; two are caused by sharp objects; two result from falls; one is due to fireworks or projectiles from air rifles, slingshots, and similar weapons; and one is caused by some small particle — dust, wood, stone, or metal — entering the eye. The major single accident that threatens blindness seems to be the fireworks-projectile category.

Many of these accidents can be prevented. Sharp and dangerous objects should be kept from children until they are sufficiently mature to use them carefully. An infant is just as likely to poke a pencil into his eye as try to write with it. Weapons such as bows and arrows, slingshots, blowguns, and rifles should neither be given to children nor placed where they can reach them.

A harried mother may sometimes let her child crawl or wander into her husband's workshop, where sharp tools or dangerous chemicals are available as fascinating toys. She may unknowingly let the infant reach into the cleaning closet where lye, ammonia, and similarly hazardous materials that could be blinding or lethal are kept. In addition to observing rules of common-sense accident prevention, parents should try to instill in the child a responsible attitude that will make him cautious regarding his own safety and that of others.

Meanwhile, children will fight, will fall, will be unable to avoid some accidents, and will continue to collect foreign substances in their eyes. A child should be made very conscious of the fact that when an eye is injured he must not rub it, or allow another child to doctor it. Instead, he should tell a parent or a teacher about the injury as quickly as possible. From that point on it remains with the adult to observe the elementary rules of first aid — with one special injunction. A child's eyes are even more vulnerable than an adult's, and therefore only a doctor should approach them — even if it is only a matter of removing a speck of dust. The only exception to this rule is when some corrosive chemical — lye or ammonia, for instance — or some burning object enters the eye. When this happens, a doctor should be called at once, and the eye should be flooded by a stream of running water for at least fifteen minutes.

Good "Seeing" Habits

Good general health is even more important to the eyes of a child than to those of an adult. It is essential to instill sound attitudes about health and hygiene in the child as early and as thoroughly as possible.

Since children generally tend to rebel against any rules of behavior that apply only to them and not to the others around them, especially their parents and siblings, they are best taught by example. The parent who warns a child against exposing his eyes to sunlight and then proceeds to sunbathe without adequately protecting his own eyes is not going to be taken very seriously.

The parent should explain to the child why his eyes are important and why they deserve special consideration. This should be done reasonably and calmly, so that the child will be able to approach the matter of eye protection with understanding, not fear.

Along with sound attitudes toward health, hygiene, and safety, the parent can help the child by teaching him to use his eyes properly, to minimize the possibility of strain.

A child's eyes are not damaged or injured in any way by reading "too much," or by reading in bed. There is no such thing as reading or using the eyes "too much"; but a real problem could be created by not using them enough. In this regard eyes are very much like muscles — improved by use, damaged by disuse. So the child's reading time should not be restricted, nor should he be limited in his television-watching time, solely in order to "preserve" his eyes.

Poor lighting, bad posture, and excessive concentration of the eyes on one spot may produce strain, fatigue, and redness regardless of what the child, or the adult for that matter, is doing. By example and by simple explanation, the parent should teach the child the importance of good posture that leaves the body comfortable and does not strain the neck muscles; of good lighting that is adequate and even, without sharp contrasts of light and shadow; and of the need to move the eyes periodically, looking away from the object being watched, so that the muscles involved in focusing the eyes are not strained by unrelieved concentration. The practice of frequently looking away from an object in order to change focus is a good one to observe no matter what we are doing and regardless of our age. This tends to relieve strain and is an effective means of "resting" the eyes.

Since children, no less than adults, seem to spend a good deal of their time watching television, it might be well to follow a few simple rules for avoiding possible strain.

Tune the station in sharply, so that the picture is as clear as possible, has a minimum of flicker, and does not have excessive contrast. If you cannot receive an acceptable picture on any channel, turn the set off until the situation can be corrected.

TV watchers should find a comfortable seat directly in front of the screen, as far away as they can get and still see the picture clearly. The screen should be as nearly eye level as possible. Watching television from the floor, as children often seem to prefer, should be discouraged, since this causes a cramped position that will fatigue the neck and eye muscles, producing strain and headache.

Illuminate the room with a soft, diffuse light that is not reflected in the television screen.

Finally, make sure that neither you nor your children stare at the picture continuously. Look away from the screen occasionally to rest your eyes.

Children are tremendously susceptible to the attitudes of their parents. This fact cannot be emphasized too strongly. If parents are careless, the children will be careless, regardless of how often or how emphatically the parents urge caution upon them. Similarly, anxious and fearful parents will provoke anxiety and fear in their children, no matter how much they try to calm them.

If a child must wear glasses, or has some ocular illness that requires special medical treatment or surgery, the parents must not allow themselves to feel that there is something strange or unusual about this, that the child is somehow inferior. The athletic father should not allow himself to feel let down because his son, due to an eye problem or some other problems, will not be able to follow in his footsteps. Nor must parents feel anxious that a daughter will be less attractive to boys because she must wear glasses. Such feelings are more than absurd — they are bound to hurt the child, not only through the outward manifestations of the parents' attitude, but, more important, by warping his own attitude toward himself.

Feelings of anxiety, apprehension, or fear are also swiftly communicated to children, no matter how the parents try to mask them. If a child must undergo medical or surgical treatment for some ocular illness or injury, it is important for the parents to adopt a matter-of-fact attitude about the situation. What the child needs at such times is calm, loving concern and support. What he does not need at all is anxiety, overconcern, and pity.

If the child must wear special glasses or a bandage, or requires continued medical treatment, his parents and others close to him should be very matter-of-fact about it. He should not be made to feel different, and neither he nor his eyes should be overprotected or given special treatment not specifically ordered by the doctor.

It may be difficult for some parents to control their own feelings sufficiently to observe these elementary rules. But if they fail to do so they are likely to provoke emotional damage that may be more serious and lasting than the original defect or injury.

4

AID FOR YOUR EYES

New Horizons for the Blind and Near-Blind   23

Only the most unthinking, unfeeling person would shrug off another's loss of sight as a condition to which he could easily adjust by dint of fortitude and willpower. Blindness is no easy prospect to face; but neither should it be considered an unmitigated disaster. The adjustments require great personal courage and, equally important, motivation. Intelligence and a full measure of adaptability are also needed, as well as understanding and moral support from family and friends.

YOUR SIGHT: FOLKLORE, FACT AND COMMON SENSE

Blindness means that the most used of all of our senses can no longer provide us with information. But this does not mean that all channels are closed. Our other senses, some only fractionally used by many of us, can be trained to open other windows upon the world. Hearing, smell, and touch can be heightened to provide much, although by no means all, of the day-to-day information we need to function.

Today the blind can "read" — with their fingers, thanks to Braille, or with their ears, by means of the newly developed "talking books." They can do productive work, support themselves, go to school, earn degrees, teach, create works of art, act, sing, play musical instruments; do a vast number of other things once considered virtually impossible to the sightless.

The completely blind person will not be able to enjoy phenomena that can only be seen — the colors of a sunset, the flight of a bird, the face of a child. But even this lack may not be irrevokable, since modern research may make it possible to "see" these things even without eyes (see chapter 26).

Many of our present attitudes regarding blindness are actually emotional responses rooted in ancient concepts. In very early times — before the development of agriculture, and even today in certain cruel environments — the blind were often left to fend for themselves. There were no food surpluses, and people literally lived from hand to mouth, each eating what he could kill or gather that day. Little if any food could be spared for those (other than infants, who mainly suckled) who did not contribute to its collection or preparation. The harsh demands of ordinary living allowed little tolerance for the aged and infirm.

Blindness was frequently considered a punishment visited by God, and the blind were pitied, shunned, or even persecuted, depending upon local and individual attitudes toward those who had incurred God's wrath. However, with Christianity making its early appeal to the multitudes of poor, oppressed, and enslaved, charity and pity for the handicapped took on a special meaning. As early as the fourth century in the city of Caesaria in Cappadocia, a region of Asia Minor, a shelter for the blind was opened by St. Basil. In the centuries that followed, many more were opened in the Near East and Europe, providing a certain measure of assistance to those "rendered helpless by the Lord."

These measures offered a degree of assistance to the blind, a far cry from earlier disregard. Nevertheless, the blind still had virtually no means of support other than charity or begging. The fact that they could develop a great number of skills, be self-supporting, and contribute to the community was not understood until relatively recently, and is still not sufficiently accepted.

For the most part this knowledge has been brought home by such exceptional individuals among the blind as John Milton, who was blind when he dictated *Paradise Lost* and *Paradise Regained*; the contemporary Cuban dancer Alicia Alonso, who though blind remains one of the world's great ballerinas; the late American pianist and entertainer Alec Templeton; Helen Keller, who was both blind and deaf.

In the United States, blindness is defined legally as the inability, even with corrective lenses, to see at twenty feet what the normal individual can see at two hundred feet; or to have a field of vision restricted to an angular distance of twenty degrees or less. Since only an estimated one fourth of all legally blind people in the United States have *no* remaining vision, it is at least theoretically possible to improve visual perception in three out of four legally blind persons.

This does not necessarily mean that the vision itself is improved. However, an increasing number of ophthalmologists believe that much of the vision remaining to the legally blind is not fully utilized, and that by training and the use of hand-held magnifying glasses and other aids, residual sight can be made more effective. To achieve this, a number of agencies for the blind have set up so-called low vision clinics. Information regarding such centers and other agencies aiding the blind is available from the American Foundation for the Blind, Inc., 15 West 16th Street, New York, N.Y. 10011.

Those who are born blind, or who lose their sight during infancy, do not have as great a problem adjusting to blindness as older children or adults who become blind. They can go to special schools, are provided with special educational materials, and since they have never known sight can — provided their parents neither overprotect nor reject them — develop into relatively well-adjusted, self-sufficient adults. A person losing his sight later in life does have adjustment problems, which may be mild, moderate, or quite serious, depending upon the individual's psychological resources and motivation.

State and private agencies provide visiting teachers to help newly blind persons over the period of early adjustment. Their job is to show the blind how they can take the path toward self-sufficiency and independence. They offer basic instruction in such tasks as dressing, cleaning, shopping, cooking, and feeding one's self — simple enough tasks for the sighted, but requiring special skills and training for the sightless.

Altogether, there are approximately four hundred government and voluntary agencies in the United States providing services to the blind. (A number of these are listed in the appendix on page 219, and the American Foundation for the Blind, Inc., provides a complete list.) These agencies offer instruction in reading and writing Braille; provide sheltered workshops where the blind can learn skills and help support themselves; give training in specialized jobs, such as taking dictation from tape recordings or directly on a typewriter. There are certain areas of work where a highly developed sense of touch or hearing may be more valuable than sight, and these may offer special opportunities for the blind. The federal government, through the Vocational Rehabilitation

Act, allocates funds which, together with state funds, are used to train blind persons for gainful employment.

The services available to the blind are many and varied. The Lighthouse, as the New York Association for the Blind is popularly known, offers an excellent example of what can and is being done by a number of similar agencies. It maintains nursery schools for blind children. It offers special home instruction for blind adults in such daily living skills as shaving, applying makeup, selecting clothes, cooking, and getting from place to place. It provides vocational training and paying jobs in its own workshop, where a number of household articles are made. It operates summer camps for blind children, adolescents, and adults. It offers recreational facilities, has a dramatic group that produces plays, a music school, a glee club, and a bowling team.

The Lighthouse also conducts low vision service clinics, where ophthalmologists seek to determine whether partially sighted adults and children can derive maximum use of their remaining vision by the use of visual aids.

Another aid to the blind, especially useful in areas of heavy automotive traffic, is the guide dog. Currently, there are approximately a dozen schools throughout the United States that provide trained dogs, and train blind persons to work with these dogs. Among these organizations are Guide Dogs for the Blind, Inc.; The Seeing Eye, Inc.; Leader Dogs for the Blind; and Guiding Eyes for the Blind, Inc. (Not all blind persons can be trained to use guide dogs, however. Since a mature sense of responsibility is necessary, as well as physical strength and stamina both for the training and the use of the dog, the very young, the elderly, and the feeble may not qualify.)

Among the most important developments giving the blind an additional window upon the world was the introduction of the Braille alphabet. Consisting of sixty-three combinations of six raised points, Braille can be read through touch. This system of reading and writing was developed in France during the first half of the nineteenth century by Louis Braille who, blinded at the age of three, evolved the alphabet from an earlier system created by Charles Barbier. Since then, a Braille method has been devised to make it possible for the blind to read musical scores, in addition to prose, poetry, and numbers.

Through the Library of Congress Division for the Blind and Physically Handicapped, a Books for the Blind program has made available thousands of books, periodicals, and musical scores printed in Braille. This material is provided to thirty-four regional libraries for the blind, which in turn, distribute it to various local public libraries.

With the advent of the long-playing record and the tape recorder, it became possible for the blind to "read" with their ears as well as with their fingers. Moreover, for the partially sighted, specially developed large-print books are now being made available through public library branches.

Lists of books, periodicals, and other materials which the blind may "read" either in Braille, or as "talking books," or in large print can be obtained without charge from the Division for the Blind, Library of Congress, Washington, D.C. 20540. Such information is also available through local or regional public libraries.

Under the Books for the Blind program, any person certified as legally blind may receive on loan from his state agency, post free and without charge, a talking book playback machine (actually a long-playing phonograph). He will then be able to borrow and play, also free of charge, any talking books available in the regional library. Books, periodicals, and other matter in Braille can be obtained through the same government-supported program.

In addition to the thirty-four regional libraries supplying reading materials to the blind, there are at present some fifty-four agencies that lend talking book machines. All told, nearly eighty thousand blind readers in the United States are currently using talking books, with approximately three thousand titles available; while more than thirteen thousand borrow books in Braille, of which six thousand or so titles are available. Among the periodicals the blind can thus read are *Reader's Digest, Newsweek, Atlantic, Harper's, Ladies' Home Journal, Good Housekeeping, Sports Illustrated, National Geographic,* and *Changing Times.*

Four major establishments in the United States produce books in Braille under government contract: Howe Press of the Perkins School for the Blind, Watertown, Massachusetts; American Printing House for the Blind, Louisville, Kentucky; Braille Institute of America, Inc., Los Angeles, California; and Clovernook Printing House for the Blind, Cincinnati, Ohio.

The two major producers of talking books are the American Printing House for the Blind in Louisville, and the American Foundation for the Blind in New York.

The books produced under the Library of Congress program are mainly recreational. However, educational materials and textbooks are recorded and circulated without charge by Recording for the Blind, Inc., New York City. Independent of the government program but cooperating with it, Recording for the Blind, Inc., makes its free service available nationally to blind elementary, high school, college, and graduate students, as well as to blind adults who require educational materials. Recorded texts are available in various fields of science, mathematics, law, computer programming, theology, and social work, etc., etc.

Large-print books and periodicals have recently proved their value as a means of providing easily read material to men, women, and children with limited vision. An increasing number of publishers are now entering this field, one of the earliest of which was National Aid to the Visually Handicapped, San Francisco, which provided books mainly for school-age children. Large-type books for adults are produced by Keith Jennison Books in New York, and by a number of other publishers via the medium of Xerox enlargement.

Thanks to these continuing advances, more and more of the world is being made available to blind people.

Eyeglasses 24

Exactly when or where eyeglasses were first used is a question that has been much argued. The Chinese made lenses from rock crystal several thousand years ago. The Egyptians and Assyrians, too, made crude lenses that had the power to magnify. One such lens, made of rock crystal, was recovered from the ruins of Nineveh, the ancient capital of Assyria. This lens, one and a half inches in diameter, was probably used about 800 B.C. Possibly some of the very fine jewelry of ancient times was made with the aid of magnifying lenses, but there is no indication that they were employed as eyeglasses serving a corrective function.

Eyeglasses were in use before the Christian era in China, but these neither magnified nor reduced the image and were designed solely, as far as is known, to treat certain illnesses. In Rome, according to the historian Pliny, Nero wore tinted glasses, with no corrective power, to shield his eyes from sunlight. He is also said to have used a magnifying lens made of an emerald.

The first recorded use of special lenses to correct failing eyesight was in thirteenth-century China, at the court of Emperor Kublai Khan. Marco Polo, a great friend and favorite of the emperor, wrote that elderly members of the court used double convex lenses to improve their diminishing vision.

The first European description of the possible use of lenses to assist or correct vision is attributed to the Franciscan scholar Roger Bacon. Because of his opposition to established dogma, Bacon was condemned to prison for fourteen years, and his work was generally ignored. Possibly in order to protect himself, Bacon wrote his scientific observations in an elaborate code. Among the writings that have been decoded by W. R. Newbold is one called *Optical Science,* which Bacon reputedly wrote just prior to his imprisonment in 1278. In this document, Bacon declared: "If a man looks at letters or other small objects through the medium of a crystal or a glass or of some other transparent body placed above the letters, and it is the smaller part of the sphere whose convexity is toward the eye, and the eye is in the air, he will see the letters much better and they will appear larger to him . . . Therefore this instrument can be useful to the aged and to those with weakened eyes. . . ."

Unfortunately, Bacon's discoveries and observations — and he made many far in advance of his time, in anatomy, medicine, physics, and other fields — were buried under the weight of ecclesiastic prohibition and never followed up.

After Bacon, a number of other Europeans referred to the use of lenses, which may or may not have been intended as eyeglasses. However, we are sure of one fact: eyeglasses were in use in Europe by the year 1352. That year the artist Thomas of Modena painted a fresco in the chapter house of Treviso in which he depicted Cardinal Hugh of Provence with eyeglasses perched on his nose.

In the fifteenth century, Gutenberg's invention of movable type and the development of cheap paper created an upsurge in the use of eyeglasses. Another spur was the great increase of trade and commerce, which brought about a widespread rise in the need for commercial records, bills of lading, inventories, and the general exchange of written communications.

All at once, it seemed, more people than ever before found themselves reading — either for pleasure, for study, or for business reasons. And people with hyperopia, who had never known they had a visual defect, realized they could not see up close very well although their middle and distance vision was perfectly adequate.

Those who needed and could afford eyeglasses swarmed to have them made. The optical industry flourished. Since it was the need to see clearly enough to read and write that compelled most people to wear eyeglasses, spectacles came to be associated with literacy, learning, and wisdom — an attitude that persists to this very day in many parts of the world.

Eyeglasses have a simple purpose — to correct defects in vision so that we can see as normally as possible. The way this is done is relatively simple in concept, but considerably more complicated in execution. The lenses of the glasses are supposed to alter the focus of the light rays that enter the eye in such a way that they will exactly compensate for the distortion caused by the defect.

In order to do this, very precise and complicated measurements must be made of the eyes. The nature of the visual disturbance — be it myopia, hyperopia, presbyopia, astigmatism — must be determined, and its extent measured. Such an examination is made by an ophthalmologist or an optometrist, both of whom are qualified to examine the eyes for defects in vision. Only the ophthalmologist, however, is medically qualified to diagnose and treat the eyes for disease and injury.

Once the examination is complete, the ophthalmologist or optometrist prescribes corrective lenses intended to balance the defect and bring eyesight back to normal. The prescribed glasses are then ground and fitted by the optometrist or by an optician, who is specially trained to grind and fit eyeglasses according to the ophthalmologist's prescription, but is not himself qualified to examine, measure, or treat the eye. In some parts of the country, the ophthalmologist does the grinding and fitting himself.

The ophthalmologist or optometrist usually begins the examination by asking about visual problems, then tests the visual acuity of each eye, and both together, with the Snellen Chart. This eye chart, which is still the standard, was developed in 1863 by Dr. Herman Snellen of the Netherlands, and is used in a number of variations for adults and children.

After the Snellen test, which helps show the furthest distance at which we can see clearly, another test determines near vision. The patient reads paragraphs printed on a card in various sizes of type, and a record is made of the smallest type he can distinguish clearly, as well as the distance at which he holds the card. This test was developed by E. Jaeger, a Viennese physician, and like the Snellen test should be used on each eye separately and both eyes together.

After these tests for near and far visual acuity, the examiner may use still another test to determine whether the light that enters the eye is properly and sharply focused on the macula lutea — the portion of the retina where visual images are supposed to be received which contains the fovea centralis, the tiny depression where vision is at its sharpest. This is the *refraction test,* and although it can be performed in several ways, the most common and possibly the most accurate is with the *retinoscope.* The patient looks directly at a beam of light projected from a mirror about three feet away. The examiner, looking through a tiny hole in the center of the mirror, studies the changes in the light beam as it is reflected back from the retina to the pupil. In this way he can determine the presence and extent of any refractive (light-bending) error in the eye, and the amount of correction needed to restore the condition to normal.

With this information on hand, the ophthalmologist or optometrist is usually able to decide the type and strength of lenses you will need to correct your vision.

Another frequently used refraction test actually allows the patient to select his own glasses. This is the *manifest refraction test* in which the examiner has the patient wear eyeglass frames with removable lenses. As he studies the eyes he keeps changing the lenses for each eye until the test chart can be seen with greatest clarity. When this point of sharpest vision for each eye is obtained, the eyes are tested together. If no problem then presents itself, the last pair of lenses is the one he will prescribe for the eyeglasses. If the patient does not see well with both eyes together, further tests will determine what additional correction is needed.

In any event, if the ophthalmologist or optometrist cannot provide lenses that will restore vision to normal in both eyes, it will be necessary to learn the specific reason. It might be a cataract, or some other disease state. A medical examination and a much more thorough eye examination will have to be performed by a qualified eye doctor, and if you have been seeing an optometrist, he will advise a visit to an ophthalmologist.

Lenses

The nearsighted or myopic person cannot see distant objects clearly, although he has no trouble whatsoever with close objects. He might be able to read the very fine print on a legal document, but be unable to recognize his wife at a distance of thirty feet.

This defect is usually due to an elongated eyeball, and the parallel light rays from distant objects have to travel further than normal to reach the retina. As a result, the light comes into sharp focus before the retina instead of on it, producing a blurred image.

Lenses to correct this condition must spread the light rays just enough to prevent their coming into focus before they reach the retina. This is accomplished by a *concave lens,* which bends the light outward just enough to compensate for the defect, making it possible for distant objects to focus directly on the retina and be seen clearly.

Since these glasses are designed only to correct for distant vision, they will create distorted images close up. Consequently, nearsighted people have to remove their glasses when reading, and put them on to recognize their wives at thirty feet or more.

Hyperopia, farsightedness, is the exact reverse of myopia. The farsighted person might recognize his wife at a distance of a hundred yards or more, but be unable to read his own name on a calling card at ordinary reading distances.

In the child and young adult, this condition is usually the result of a shorter than normal eyeball which, while presenting no problem when seeing distant objects, causes close objects to look blurred. Light from these objects, though refracted normally by the lens, is not yet in focus by the time it reaches the retina, for the simple reason that the retina is too close.

In middle-aged or older people, this condition may have

another cause — the progressive inability of the lens of the eye to accommodate for close vision, presbyopia.

To correct the defect in either case, a lens is needed that will bend the light rays toward each other just enough to bring them into focus on the retina. In the hyperopic young person, this will compensate for the fact that the retina is closer to the front of the eye than normally; in the presbyopic older person, it will compensate for the declining ability of the eye's lens to bend the light from close objects.

The corrective lens used for this purpose is *convex*. Astigmatism is a much more complex problem than either nearsightedness or farsightedness. Not only may either of these be present and need correction, but an additional problem is caused by an unevenness of the lens or cornea. Because of this unevenness, not all of the rays of light entering the eye are bent equally. As a result, the image focused on the retina is somewhat distorted.

In order to correct for this distortion, the ophthalmologist or optometrist must first determine the plane of the defect. It might be horizontal, vertical, or oblique. Once this has been established by proper tests, the defect can be corrected with a *cylindrical lens* — one that is a section of a cylinder rather than a sphere. This type of lens is designed to bend light only in the plane of the defect, compensating for the particular astigmatic distortion causing the problem.

Assume that you are slightly myopic and have been wearing glasses to correct your nearsightedness since school days. You are now approaching the age of fifty and notice that it is becoming increasingly difficult to see near objects very clearly without glasses.

You go to the eye doctor and tell him what the problem is. He tests your eyes and tells you that, in addition to the myopia, you now have developed presbyopia and will need glasses to see close objects clearly.

The choice you have, then, is to use two different pairs of glasses, changing from one to the other depending upon the distance of the object you are looking at; or take advantage of Benjamin Franklin's ingenuity and wear a single pair of *bifocal glasses* for near *and* distant vision.

Franklin, who was among other things a man of great common sense, did not see why it was necessary to put up with the nuisance of constantly having to change glasses. So he had the lenses of his two pairs of glasses cut in half. Then, combining the top half from a distance-correction lens with the bottom half of a close-correction lens, he had these combination lenses fitted into a single pair of eyeglass frames.

The results were completely satisfactory. As Franklin wrote to his friend George Whately in 1785: "By this means, as I wear my spectacles constantly, I have only to move my eyes up or down, as I want to see distinctly far or near, the proper glasses being always ready. This I find more particularly convenient."

Modern techniques of glassmaking and fusing have permitted vast improvements over the original bifocals conceived by Benjamin Franklin, but the delightful simplicity of the idea remains unchanged. It has been estimated that of every one hundred people who develop presbyopia, only four will be able to do with simple reading glasses. The other ninety-six will have some additional defect that will make two or more sets of eyeglasses necessary. For many of them, this product of Franklin's genius is received as a blessing.

Because a period of adjustment is sometimes necessary before most people can become accustomed to bifocals, they may seem difficult and even annoying to wear at first. Some people never become used to them. But for the majority, the comfort and convenience is apparent almost at once.

This is especially true of people whose work makes them shift their eyes rapidly between near and distant objects. A surveyor, for example, has to read and make entries on a map, which requires close vision, then look for markers which may be a considerable distance away. A photographer has to take close-up readings on his light meter and make adjustments on his camera, then look at the subject, who is too far away to be seen clearly with the same glasses. There are countless similar situations, both at work and at play, in which life would be much more complicated without bifocal lenses.

There are cases in which middle vision is also affected, requiring three separate prescriptions. A modification of Franklin's idea has been developed to deal with this problem as well — *trifocal lenses*. Trifocals are made in three segments, one above the other, the lowest section for close-up seeing, the next higher for middle distance, and the topmost for seeing distant objects. Thanks to this type of lens, defects can be corrected over the whole range of vision, and the function of the eyes restored to as nearly normal a condition as possible. Using trifocal lenses, a factory foreman, for instance, would be able to read a production schedule, examine a machine some ten feet away, and watch a delivery at the other end of the floor without having to change eyeglasses.

An important feature of almost every pair of eyeglasses is the frame into which the lenses are set. These should be properly fitted and adjusted to each individual's needs. Improperly fitted glasses can be uncomfortable, spoil our appearance, and, much more important, prevent us from seeing as clearly as we should.

Eyeglasses are used to correct a number of other conditions that produce abnormal vision. An example is *aniseikonia*, in which the image pattern on one retina differs in size and shape from the image pattern on the other. Because of the effort of the brain to attempt to fuse the images, a number of associated disturbances are produced, such as headaches, nervous tension, and occasionally disorders of the digestive system.

Valuable though eyeglasses may be in the practical correction of ocular disturbances, they are not the ideal solution, at least not in theory.

The eye, after all, is a self-contained optical system that moves almost constantly. As the eyeball moves, all of the elements within it move and continuously adjust to the changing scene. Thus the lens within the eye also moves and adjusts, correcting focus to meet each new demand. When eyeglasses are used, a fixed and immovable element is added to this system. These corrective lenses do not move with the eyeballs as do the natural lenses. In some troublesome conditions this is a distinct fault.

Ideally, the best solution would be to substitute a workable lens for the eye's crystalline lens. Experiments along these lines are already under way.

The next best solution would be to attach a lens to the eye itself, one that would move with the eyeball. Such a lens is already in use — the *contact lens*.

Contact Lenses 25

An estimated ~~ten~~ 15 (1980) million Americans are currently wearing contact lenses. Made of shatterproof plastic and greatly improved in recent years, in many instances they are extremely practical.

Contact lenses are not a particularly new idea; yet they represent one of the most recent advances in vision correction. The principle of the contact lens was described by Sir John Herschel in 1827, but the first usable series of such lenses did not appear upon the market until 1911. And it was not until 1948 that the contact lens designed for the individual cornea was conceived, by Kevin Tuohy. Seven years later, in 1955, this had finally been developed to the point where it could be placed in general use.

The idea of the contact lens as suggested by Herschel was extremely simple and logical. It consisted of attaching a lens made of glass to the eye itself, but the lens lay in front of the cornea instead of behind it. Today, these lenses are made of plastic.

Actually, the plastic surface of the contact lens itself takes over the function of the cornea. Through surface tension the contact lens floats upon the eye on a layer of lacrimal fluid which, by filling the open space behind the curved lens surface, becomes a liquid portion of the lens.

Two general types of contact lenses are used to correct defects in vision: the *scleral lens,* which covers the entire exposed surface of the eye, and the *corneal lens,* which covers just the cornea. A third type of contact lens has recently been developed, not to correct vision but to help treat certain corneal diseases. This is the *flush-fitting scleral lens.*

In most cases contact lenses are at least as effective as ordinary eyeglasses in correcting defects in vision, and in many instances are superior. By moving with the eye, the lens maintains the same relative relationship to the retina that the normal crystalline lens would. Contact lenses provide a clearer field of vision, since they eliminate the need for eyeglass frames. They also seem to be more effective than eyeglasses in correcting the irregularities of the cornea that cause astigmatism.

A disadvantage of the contact lens is that it can only effectively correct for a single error. In the person with both presbyopia and myopia, for instance, the contact lens could correct the myopia but reading glasses would be necessary to compensate for the presbyopia. This particular disadvantage may be overcome by the perfection of bifocal type contact lenses. These are being tested experimentally, but have not yet proved satisfactory.

Generally, the greatest advantage of contact lenses over standard eyeglasses is in extreme cases of myopia, astigmatism, and hyperopia. They are also, for the present at least, the best

CONTACT LENSES

substitute for a cataractous lens that has been removed. For this use, they may be replaced by implanted plastic lenses in the not too distant future.

Another use to which contact lenses are occasionally put is in the correction of certain cases of near blindness. In some extreme cases, only eyeglasses so thick as to be unwearable would make vision possible. A combination of contact lenses and eyeglasses can often provide a wearable solution.

The best reason for wearing contact lenses is that they may be the most effective means of correcting a particular visual defect. There are a number of other reasons, almost equally good.

Contact lenses are especially useful for actors or other performers whose roles may not allow them to wear eyeglasses. Contact lenses usually will not be dislodged by running, jumping, or similar activity, and so can be worn with good effect by football, baseball, basketball, and hockey players, runners, skiers, acrobats, and so on. However, contact lenses should not be worn by swimmers, because the lenses may float away when the eyes are open under water.

Contact lenses might also be worn to good advantage by people who must do extremely sensitive work under certain difficult conditions. They would prove a great boon, for instance, under circumstances where eyeglasses might steam up, ice up, or be covered by snow. If both hands are occupied at the time, the wearer of eyeglasses can be left temporarily blind.

To a large extent, contact lenses are also worn for cosmetic reasons. Some people feel that eyeglasses spoil their appearance and prefer the less obvious contact lenses. This may not seem to be the best reason for wearing them, but it is certainly a valid one, particularly if it helps preserve an individual's self-confidence.

Apart from the fact that some visual defects may not be correctable with contact lenses, there are a number of other possible reasons why eyeglasses might be preferable in some instances.

First of all, there are people who simply cannot tolerate having any foreign substance on their eyes. These people find it impossible to wear contact lenses. Some people can tolerate them only for a limited period of time, and then must remove them to rest the eyes. This period of tolerance differs with the individual, but practically everyone who wears scleral contact lenses will need a rest period, during which he will probably wear eyeglasses. Corneal contact lenses are usually better tolerated.

The insertion of contact lenses into the eyes requires a certain amount of skill and manual dexterity which some people do not possess. People with diseases that cause tremor or unsteadiness, Parkinson's disease for example, would obviously be unable to manage contact lenses. Unless contact lenses are expertly fitted and properly placed they can irritate the eye, and in some cases cause serious damage.

Expense is another possible disadvantage, since contact lenses are substantially more costly than eyeglasses. Furthermore, they are very easy to lose and very difficult to find.

The National Society for the Prevention of Blindness urges that contact lenses be ordered only after an ophthalmologist has given his approval. He will determine whether such lenses will be suitable to correct the visual disturbance and, further, the possible degree of difficulty the patient may have in wearing them. Under no circumstances should a person decide upon contact lenses for himself, or have them fitted by anyone whose professional competence is not fully assured — regardless of how dazzlingly high or temptingly low the cost may be.

The corneal lens is the most popular type in the world today, with an estimated nine to ten million people presently wearing them in the United States alone. The most modern of the contact lenses, it is generally the most effective and the easiest to wear.

Each lens has to be specially designed for the individual eye. It fits only over the cornea, held in place by the surface tension of the thin film of tears on which it floats, and it must fit the curve of the cornea precisely.

Dr. Louis J. Girard of Baylor University in Houston, Texas, one of the acknowledged authorities on contact lenses, explains the need for such exact custom fitting thus: "The optical zone of the cornea can vary tremendously from one individual to another, and may also vary from one eye to another."

Extremely precise measurements have to be made of the front curvature of the cornea. If there were no other reason, this alone would dictate the need to have the job done only by a fully competent specialist.

The refractive or light-bending aspects of the lens, designed to correct a particular visual defect, are ground on the outer surface. This, in turn, helps determine the overall thickness of the contact lens. However, the thickness of each lens is kept to the absolute minimum that is allowable to maintain its stability, since added thickness seems to produce added discomfort.

After the corneal lens has been ground, polished, and fitted, the ophthalmologist or optometrist will check it and make whatever adjustments are necessary to provide for maximum comfort and vision correction.

Dr. Girard says: "Such custom-designed corneal lenses have proven to be successful in 90 to 95 percent of the people fitted. They are tolerated all of the wearer's waking hours, and require additional modification in only 50 percent of the cases."

Moreover, assuming that they have been properly fitted and the person wearing them handles them properly, these lenses should cause no damage to the eye.

The scleral lens is the oldest of the contact types. It was first blown from glass in 1887 by F. A. Muller, but could not be particularly useful until a way was found to fit such a lens properly. This was finally achieved in 1938, when a technique was developed for making an impression of the eye in a mold, reproducing it in a plastic material.

The section of this plastic lens over the cornea was then hollowed out and an optical surface ground onto the area. This chamber between the inner surface of the contact lens and the outer surface of the cornea was filled with a buffered salt solution. The lens was then placed over the whole of the forward portion of the eye and fitted under the eyelids.

Because this early type of scleral lens blocked the flow of tears from the lacrimal gland, it was not possible to wear it for more than a few hours at a time. Today, although the design of the scleral lens remains basically the same, channels have been built into it to permit the circulation of tears.

When the scleral lens is fitted today, an anesthetic is applied to the eye and a very soft, jellylike material used to make a smooth impression. A cast is then prepared from this impression, and the lens is made from the cast. The proper refractive correction required by the eye is then ground on the forward surface of the plastic lens.

The scleral lens, although it was the first of the contact lenses, is not particularly popular today, especially since it can only be worn for a limited time before it must be removed to rest the eye. However, it is useful in certain conditions where a corneal lens cannot be used.

The flush-fitting scleral lens is not used at all for visual correction, but as an aid to healing. It is molded to fit flush against the contour of the eye, separated from the cornea only by a layer of tears.

"One of the most exciting developments in contact lenses and even in ophthalmology," Dr. Girard reported to a meeting of

Research to Prevent Blindness, Inc., in 1965, "has been the development of the flush-fitting scleral lens for the treatment of certain corneal diseases."

Dr. Girard and his associates at Baylor University had used this type of lens on approximately one hundred patients at the time he made the report. Many of them had suffered alkali burns of the cornea, chronic ulcerations, mustard gas burns, and a number of other potentially blinding conditions such as severe inflammations, infections, and so on. In a number of these cases, said Dr. Girard, the results have been excellent, with the cornea healing and vision restored. For this reason, he said, the use of the flush-fitting scleral lens has become the "treatment of choice" in some of the conditions.

As more and more people wear contact lenses, the latent dangers become more apparent. We have already noted that poorly designed or badly fitted lenses can irritate, inflame, and damage the cornea. If the person wearing the lens is highly motivated, he may sometimes be able to tolerate it despite the poor fit. There is also good evidence that the cornea may become less sensitive after wearing a contact lens. Nevertheless, badly fitted and poorly designed lenses are a potential hazard. Nor is there any good reason why anyone should endure unnecessary discomfort.

Another danger arises from simple human folly. Some people wearing contact lenses forget to remove them at bedtime. Or perhaps they are careless about cleaning the lens properly, which can result in serious injury or infection.

There have also been instances of corneal ulcers developing in patients with corneal lenses. No scientific investigation of the subject has been undertaken as yet, so it remains to be established whether such corneal ulcers result from the wearing of the lenses, or from their misuse.

The growing use of contact lenses, although still largely for cosmetic reasons, has stimulated a new research which has already borne fruit in the flush-fitting lens. Other advances are expected. A number of universities have followed the lead taken by Baylor University to include the subject of contact lenses in their curriculum, which will greatly stimulate research and progress.

The contact lens is by no means perfect, and many problems remain to be solved before the ideal lens is finally evolved. But with the cooperation of the practicing ophthalmologist and optometrist, the university teacher, and the basic scientist, such an ideal lens is a distinct possibility.

Eyes on the Future   26

The opacity of cataracts was recognized thousands of years ago, and even treated rationally by the Egyptians, Chinese, and Hindus; but the subtler causes of blindness, such as circulatory or nervous disorders, metabolic disturbances like diabetes, hereditary defects, bacterial and viral infections, could only be recognized after we had developed the background and technology necessary to identify the diseases and trace their relationships to the eyes.

Without the invention of the microscope, for instance, it would have been impossible to recognize that microbes are a cause of infection. Without the ophthalmoscope that made the retina available for examination, it would have been impossible to see the degenerative changes in the tiny blood vessels of the retina caused by diabetes, high blood pressure, and the attrition of aging.

Similarly, effective treatment of ocular disease and visual disturbances is, with few exceptions, a fairly recent development. Eyeglasses have been in use for several hundred years, but the instruments required to make adequate tests of the precise nature and extent of vision loss are relatively new. And without them it was impossible to make fully satisfactory correction.

The sulfa drugs, most antibiotics, and the anti-inflammatory drugs are all products of recent times. Until they were made available, many diseases that are now routinely cured were fundamentally untreatable and almost invariably caused blindness. Surgery, too, has made great advances in recent years. New techniques, equipment, anesthetics, and drugs make it possible to perform operations that were previously impossible. Most important of all the advances, however, has been the growing understanding of the nature of the diseases that affect our vision and how this related to the body as a whole.

Basic research has opened many new areas with its probing questions, and many of the answers are being used to explore still newer areas.

By what process is light energy converted into nerve energy in the retina? How is this nerve energy interpreted by the brain to cause a definite image to be imprinted upon our consciousness? What is the nature of the autoimmune process and exactly how and why do parts of our own bodies turn upon other parts? Precisely which hereditary factors influence our vision, and by what means can our genetic makeup be changed so that possible defects are eliminated?

The rate at which scientists are finding answers to such questions seems to multiply each year. There are more scientists and researchers alive today than existed throughout all of man's time on earth until the dawn of the twentieth century, and advances are taking place in the whole range of human endeavor — physics, chemistry, engineering, the development of new materials, new instruments. Each advance in one area helps provide the substance for advances in other areas — so the process spirals upward.

Contact lenses became practical only in the 1960's, mainly because of the development of effective plastics.

The use of fluorescent dyes, which can be injected into the bloodstream, allows us to photograph the retinal capillaries with a motion picture camera combining the features of a microscope and ophthalmoscope. In this way we can see what happens to these blood vessels in various disease states and, in turn, anticipate what damage may be done to the retina by diseases in other parts of the body.

Progress in ophthalmology spurs progress in the field of internal medicine. Examination of the eyes now can provide early clues to the presence of disease elsewhere — diabetes, hypertension, circulatory disturbances, tumors, anemia, leukemia, glandular and metabolic malfunctions, and so on.

Cataract Prevention

Whatever the cause of cataracts, the result is a series of chemical events that make the lens turn opaque. If these events were better understood, it would then be possible, at least theoretically, to stop their progress and thus prevent cataract formation or, conceivably, to stop the progress of the cataract by some medical means. This problem is being studied in a number of laboratories both in the United States and abroad.

Some cataracts are known to be associated with diabetes, a disease in which there is an inability to use the sugar, *glucose;* and with the genetic defect in children known as *galactosemia,* in which a child is unable to utilize *galactose,* another form of sugar.

Furthermore, cataracts can be produced in experimental animals by feeding them still another form of sugar, *xylose*.

From these observations, it would seem that high concentrations of sugar in the aqueous humor may cause the lens to become opaque. So far, scientists have offered two possible explanations. Dr. Jin Kinoshita of Harvard suggests that these sugars, which are known to be converted into sugar alcohols in the lens, set into motion a process whereby the lens absorbs fluids. This causes the lens fibers to swell, then burst and disintegrate, resulting in the cataract.

A second possible explanation, put forward by Drs. V. Everett Kinsey and D. V. N. Reddy of Wayne State University in Detroit, is based on experiments showing that when high concentrations of sugar were present in rats, the amount of free amino acids — the building blocks of protein — was reduced about 90 percent.

"Could it be," asks Dr. Kinsey, "that a lack of amino acids needed for the resynthesis of proteins in the lens causes it to become opaque?"

It is still too early for definite conclusions to be reached regarding the actual mechanism of cataract formation, but already several new lines of research suggest themselves. "For instance," says Dr. Kinsey, "a search might be made for a means of inhibiting the enzyme that is responsible for converting sugars to sugar alcohols."

Another possible area for exploration is the development of a dietary approach that might increase the levels of amino acids in the blood and thus perhaps prevent or delay the appearance of "sugar" cataracts.

Although specially designed, lightweight plastic lenses are now used by many persons who have had their crystalline lenses removed because of cataract, there is still considerable room for improvement, and contact lenses are not suitable for everyone.

Such people can, of course, wear corrective eyeglasses. But these, unfortunately, have to employ thick lenses, and may be considered too uncomfortable and disturbing for sustained wear. Of course, some vision is possible in the eye after the cataract has been removed, even without a corrective lens. And if the other eye is in good condition, it often is not essential to attempt to correct the vision in the operated eye.

A new approach to the problem of restoring vision may make these questions academic. Instead of placing a lens over the eye or in front of it, scientists are experimenting with the possibility of implanting a plastic lens in the space from which the cataractous lens has been removed. This would allow for the restoration of a condition much closer to the normal state than is possible with either contact lenses or eyeglasses. Several attempts to achieve this have already been made, but the process has not yet been developed to a point where it can be considered safe or practical. Nevertheless, the possibilities are encouraging and the work is continuing with constantly improving materials, designs, and techniques.

Plastic Replacements for Diseased Corneas

The transplantation of corneal tissue from a donor eye is not always successful. These grafts sometimes become opaque or are heavily infiltrated by blood vessels, making useful vision impossible. There has recently been an upsurge of interest in an idea that is more than a century old — the use of artificial corneas for transplantation. The earliest experimental implants were made of glass, and these were soon pushed out from the eye. Recently, with the development of new types of inert plastics and other materials, the possibilities have improved considerably.

The artificial cornea is designed to replace the diseased section, fitting precisely and constructed to provide the correct curvature needed for normal vision. It is then fastened into place surgically, by the surgeon using an operating microscope to do the delicate work required.

In 1965, Dr. Arthur Gerard DeVoe of Columbia University presented a progress report at a seminar in ophthalmology organized by Research to Prevent Blindness, Inc. "At the present state of our knowledge," he said, "we are employing the implant only in eyes that are otherwise hopelessly lost — eyes that have had multiple tissue transplants that failed, and eyes in which we know from previous experience that corneal transplantation is doomed to failure.

"In some of these individuals we have been able to give reading vision, as well as distance vision in the order of 20/25 for periods up to about four years."

These results convince Dr. DeVoe that further trial with this technique is justified. However, he does not believe that this operation should be performed at this stage on someone who has normal vision in one eye, or for whom the chance of successful corneal tissue transplantation is good.

New Techniques for Earlier Disease Detection

Early diagnosis may not be of great value in managing cataract, but in glaucoma, uveitis, retinal disease, choroid inflammations, and tumors it may prevent serious loss of vision.

Recently, scientists have developed a new approach to glaucoma detection. This test may not only indicate the presence of the disease before any other presently available, but can also show whether an individual may be susceptible to glaucoma and likely to develop it in the future. In addition to making early treatment possible, glaucoma prevention becomes a very real prospect.

The test is based on the observation that the steroid drugs, such as cortisone and its chemical cousins, while excellent in treating certain inflammations, allergic conditions, and autoimmune diseases, also impose several possible hazards. For one thing, when applied to the eye directly, they tend to raise the fluid pressure within the eye temporarily in persons with glaucoma, in whom this pressure is already elevated. Obviously, then, these drugs should be avoided by people who have overt glaucoma. But the steroid disadvantage may be turned to advantage if it can be used to test people whose glaucoma is so mild that it is still undetectable, or in those who are genetically likely to develop glaucoma some time in the future. Should the application of steroid drugs to the eyes of these people result in a temporary rise in pressure, and if this is clearly associated with the later development of glaucoma, then the value of this test will have been established.

Other scientists in a number of research centers are expanding another line of research that is leading to earlier diagnosis of a number of ocular disturbances. This is the use of *fluorescein,* a fluorescent dye. Injected into the bloodstream, this dye permits rapid-sequence photographs as well as motion pictures to be taken of the blood flow as it glows in the vessels of the retina, choroid, and optic nerve. Using this method, doctors have been able to chart the characteristic changes that take place in these blood vessels as a consequence of various disease states.

With this information, doctors are able to spot diabetic retinopathy, sometimes even before the presence of diabetes itself is suspected; they can see the early and late changes of hypertensive retinopathy and follow the effects of treatment; they can tell the difference between malignant and benign tumors of the eye; they can locate obstructions in blood vessels that might lead to serious damage to vision; they can determine whether the retina or choroid is affected by disease — a very important distinction which is often difficult to make and which may have a profound effect upon the success of treatment.

Fluorescein is not the only material being tried to permit diagnostic inspection of the blood flow to and in the eye. Currently, experiments are being conducted using radioactive isotopes that are measured as they pass through the vessels of the eye. Other researchers are employing highly sensitive devices to meter the flow of blood through the ophthalmic artery; still others are experimenting with instruments able to detect minute variations in the light reflected from the retinal area.

All these research projects are designed to increase our understanding of what happens within the eye before, during, and after the onset of disease. With this knowledge, earlier detection and better treatment are made possible, and prevention may even become feasible in some presently unpreventable conditions.

Experiments currently being conducted at Georgetown University in Washington, D.C., if successful, lead to improvements in the treatment of ocular tumors, uveitis, and infection of the eye. Scientists there are attempting to isolate the eye by what is called a *cannulation-perfusion technique.*

Eyes donated to research are placed in an environment that provides them with certain nutrients and other substances, under rigid control. A drug is introduced into the environment and the effects upon the isolated eye are then studied. In this way, it is hoped, the Georgetown scientists will be able to judge with great accuracy the therapeutic value of drugs already being used, and to test the possible value of the newer experimental drugs as they are developed.

Adverse Effects of Some Drugs

While some researchers are attempting to find better drugs for the treatment of ocular disease, others are looking into the possibility that some drugs, used for other conditions, may be harmful to the eyes.

During the last few years, a vast number of new drugs have been developed for the treatment of many ills. Some of these, such as the antibiotics, may save life in a number of situations; yet these same drugs, under other circumstances, may be actually harmful. Not only that, but two drugs that can be administered separately with great benefit might produce a harmful effect if administered together.

(For this reason, incidentally, it is important for people not to attempt self-medication, and to let their doctors know of any drug allergy they may have and whether they are taking any drugs that he has not prescribed.)

An increasing amount of research is being directed into the possibly harmful side effects of some drugs, and into the likelihood of two harmless drugs interacting to produce an unlooked-for damaging action.

Certain drugs, such as chloraquin, used to treat malaria and rheumatoid arthritis, may be damaging to the retina and cornea unless used with great care. Phenothiazine derivatives, used as tranquilizers, may also produce harmful changes to the eye.

Vitamins, too, carry a hazard — not only in their absence but in excess. Vitamin A deficiency, for instance, is known to result in a decline in visual acuity and in night blindness. Yet taken in excessive amounts, this vitamin or vitamin D may provoke the development of corneal opacities.

Changing Defective Heredity

Many of the problems that affect vision are known to be inherited. Also inherited is an increase in susceptibility to certain diseases. Myopia, hyperopia, astigmatism, and color blindness are, for the most part, due to defects that are passed along from generation to generation. Glaucoma and cataracts as well often have a genetic component.

There are also systemic and metabolic diseases that produce an incidental effect upon vision. Many of these are related to genetic susceptibility. Diabetes, associated with retinopathy and cataract formation, is a classic example.

These defects are handed down from one generation to another through the germ cells of the parents. If the gene, through mutation or other accident, is abnormal, then the cells or activity that result will be abnormal. If the gene is missing, another abnormality will be produced.

Such researchers as Sir Archibald E. Carrod and Nobel Laureates Edward L. Tatum, George W. Beadle, and Joshua Lederberg have tried to pinpoint the manner in which the gene actually causes abnormality. They have found that each gene is directly related to the creation of a specific enzyme. Enzymes are biochemical catalysts — they regulate chemical activity within the body — and each enzyme is involved in only a single action. If it is missing or inactive, no other enzyme can normally step in and take over.

Where a genetic defect exists, the scientists found, it arises because an abnormal or missing gene results in an abnormal or missing enzyme. This, in turn, brings about a failure in the normal chemistry in the body.

Of course, genetic abnormalities are considerably more complicated than this brief explanation indicates. No gene, for instance, acts completely by itself, but is influenced by a multitude of factors that exist in its environment.

The chromosomes — the microscopic filaments that serve as gene-carrying bundles within each cell — are also subject to change. In mongolism, a form of mental retardation that is associated with a number of eye defects such as cataracts and strabismus, scientists have found an abnormality in the number of chromosomes. In the normal human, each body cell contains forty-six chromosomes — twenty-three from each of the parents. But the mongoloid usually has forty-seven.

For a long time it was believed that very little if anything could be done about genetic defects. Now, with scientists learning how to identify the particular gene-enzyme abnormality, they are able to compensate for the breakdown in biochemical activity in a growing number of situations.

Such inborn errors of metabolism as *galactosemia* and *phenylketonuria* (PKU), which produce mental retardation and ocular problems in infants, can, if detected early enough, be prevented from doing damage. This is achieved by regulating the diet in such a way as to compensate for the enzyme defect. However, this is only an indirect approach to the problem. It does not attempt to correct the defect by replacing the missing or abnormal enzyme.

Currently there is a growing wave of interest in the whole question of genetic regulation and modification. Some scientists are even predicting that the present "nuclear age" will soon be supplanted by the "genetic age."

Attempts are being made, experimentally, to learn how enzyme formation can be stimulated or how defective enzymes and even genes might be altered and restored to normal.

Only a few years ago the very idea of correcting defective heredity might have seemed inconceivable. Today it is a major goal of intensive research. Although no success has yet been reported, the implications of this work are so vast and reach out in so many directions that they are literally beyond calculation.

Stimulation of Vision

One of the reasons why amblyopia and some other defects in vision have not been clearly understood is that there has been no effective way of studying them. Recent developments are changing this, especially the new techniques that can measure the electrical activity of different parts of the nervous system.

At Harvard University, Drs. David Hubel and Torsten Wiesel implanted microelectrodes — tiny devices designed to pick up electrical impulses indicative of nerve activity — in different parts of the visual systems of immature experimental animals. Some of these animals were deprived of normal visual stimulation, and others were allowed to use their eyes normally.

The results were very exciting to the scientists. In the deprived animals it was found that actual changes involving both structure and function had taken place in parts of the brain involved in the visual process.

Similar experiments are presently being conducted by Dr. von Noorden at the Wilmer Institute of Johns Hopkins University. By depriving monkeys and other primates of the visual stimulus of light and form, he hopes to arrive at a better understanding of how amblyopia is produced and how it causes loss of vision. Once these mechanisms are clarified, Dr. von Noorden hopes "this will enable us in due time to improve our methods of treatment and prevention."

The fact that stimulation or use improves most activity and that lack of stimulation retards it has been shown in so many different areas that it is almost a truism. Exercising muscles or mental processes — learning, memory, or imagination — will improve them. Inactivity will cause deterioration. This is apparently also true of seeing, which involves muscles as well as nervous and mental processes.

This apparently applies even to people with initially normal vision, as the Navy learned when its new atomic submarines made submerged voyages for prolonged periods. The men in the submarines, living and working in close quarters where distant vision was not only unnecessary but impossible, developed a form of myopia. Apparently, because the muscular and other elements involved in distant seeing received no stimulation from use, they simply deteriorated and left the men nearsighted.

One would reasonably expect that this type of damage could be corrected by restimulation and retraining, but it might not be if the damage has endured long enough to produce permanent changes.

The implications of this are most interesting. If lack of stimulation dulls otherwise good vision, could planned and directed stimulation make good vision even better?

On the face of it, the answer to this question would be "no." The eye is an optical system with specific characteristics, and it cannot do better than the optimum possible to that system. Photographers, for instance, might improve with practice, but their cameras will not. For the camera to produce better pictures it would need either a new and improved optical system, or a more capable photographer.

Assuming that we cannot change our eyes, can we possibly improve the photographer — the portion of the brain that directs the eye and interprets its data?

One of the puzzling facts about vision is that two people whose eyes are apparently identical, according to all of the available tests, often show distinct differences in how well they see.

Not only do some people see better than others with equal vision, but each one of us can see certain things better than other things even though they may be the same size and distance from us.

A good example of this is that we can recognize close friends at measurably greater distances than mere acquaintances. We do not see them more clearly, but we do perceive them more distinctly.

The reason for this lies in the fact that visual perception depends upon matching what our eyes see against information already stored in our brains — data derived from experience, intellect, imagination, and other sources. This combination of "seen" clues — pertaining to size, shape, color, motion and configuration — combined with the so-called mental factors, gives us our visual perception.

The more clues we receive through our eyes, the less mental data is needed to tell us what we are seeing. And conversely, the more mental data we have, the fewer visual clues are needed. Consequently, we do not have to see a friend as clearly as an acquaintance to recognize him. A blur of motion through a stand of trees can be identified as a bird, although we do not actually "see" it.

The ability to perceive the theoretically unseeable is not new to science, but its details still baffle the scientists. Major Gordon Cooper, when he was one hundred miles in space, reported seeing a car on a dusty road, and a railroad train. Other astronauts have reported seeing the wakes of ships and other objects. Yet none of these could be seen if we consider the optical qualities of the human eye. The human eye simply cannot see those things at those distances. But they were perceived.

Similar impossibilities have been confirmed in the laboratory by a number of scientists, including Dr. W. Bruce Clark of the Nicollet Clinic in Minneapolis.

"Some of these capabilities that have been demonstrated in the laboratory are truly amazing and some appear to be optically and physiologically 'impossible,'" he says. "From what we know about the optics of the human eye, we know with certainty that resolution at the retina is not good enough to explain these human capabilities. Likewise, we know that the size of the retinal cone mosaic is a bit too coarse to explain the perceivable detail, even if the optics were perfect."

Evaluating all of the known factors, Dr. Clark is convinced that the average man rarely uses his visual capacity fully. But with proper motivation and specific visual training it is now believed that a highly intelligent, experienced man in good functional health can be conditioned to perceive visually what might ordinarily be beyond the capacity of his eyes to see.

Eyeless Sight

Even seeing without eyes has also moved into the realm of possibility. This seemingly revolutionary prospect was brought closer by the development of an electronic device that picks up light signals and sends their impulses directly to the brain. In effect it replaces the eyes.

The instrument, called the *amauroscope*, was developed by a research team headed by Dr. Armando del Campo, professor of psychiatry at the National University of Mexico. Consisting of photoelectric cells and other electronic equipment fitted into a container about the size and shape of a skin diver's mask, the amauroscope fits over the eyes. Light falling upon it excites the cells into sending out a pattern of electrical impulses, which are conducted to a number of sites around the eye and behind the ear where they can stimulate nerves involved in sending visual messages to the brain. The wires carrying these impulses are not implanted, but are fastened to the surface of the skin.

In effect, what the amauroscope attempts to do is very like what is done by the eyes. It perceives patterns of light signals, converts them into electrical impulses, and sends them to the brain for interpretation. At this stage, Dr. del Campo believes that at least two more years will be needed before a practical model will become available. But tests with scores of blind people have already suggested amazing possibilities. One man of thirty-six, blind for twenty-seven years and without eyeballs, has been shown in a filmed experiment to find his way through an obstacle course while wearing the amauroscope. He walked around a number of objects and people in his path, seeing them only as dark shadows against a light field but able to perceive their position and distance, thus avoiding collisions.

So far, the amauroscope is only capable of distinguishing light and shadow. It cannot differentiate the finer gradations that make it possible to see details.

In an experiment with both blind subjects and blindfolded subjects who could otherwise see normally, it was possible with the amauroscope to perceive a cigarette lighter's flame, a candlelight, the shadow of an object, hand, or person passing in front of the face. Blind people wearing the amauroscope have even been able to eat at a table set with white tableware on a dark tablecloth.

In two years' time, the Mexican scientist hopes, the device will be developed sufficiently to be capable of detecting light signals from a distance of about twenty-five feet and be able to distinguish some additional detail — "perhaps have the visual capability of an insect's eyes."

Man's curiosity and genius are indeed reaching out into many new and previously unexplored regions. Newer and more effective ways of preventing blindness and improving vision are being discovered, and even the blind, themselves, may be allowed to see.

APPENDIX

BIBLIOGRAPHY

GLOSSARY

INDEX

Appendix

National Agencies and Organizations Serving to Prevent Blindness and Help the Blind (Partial List)

Federal Agencies

Library of Congress, Division for the Blind and Physically Handicapped, Washington, D.C. 20540
   Provides and distributes books in Braille and talking books as part of national program to bring free reading materials to the blind.

APPENDIX

National Institute of Neurological Diseases and Blindness, Bethesda, Maryland 20014
> Conducts and supports research into the causes and prevention of blindness, treatment of eye diseases.

Office of Education, Department of Health, Education and Welfare, Washington, D.C. 20202
> Provides consultative services to school systems for the development of educational programs for blind and otherwise handicapped children.

Veterans' Administration, Washington, D.C. 20420
> Provides medical and hospital care, rehabilitation, economic assistance to blinded veterans.

Vocational Rehabilitation Administration, Division of Services to the Blind, Department of Health, Education and Welfare, Washington, D.C. 20201
> Assists state agencies develop programs of vocational rehabilitation, employment expansion, and commercial ventures for the blind.

Welfare Administration, Bureau of Family Services, Department of Health, Education and Welfare, Washington, D.C. 20201
> Helps the states provide financial and other assistance to the needy blind.

Consultative Voluntary Agencies

American Foundation for the Blind, Inc., 15 West 16th Street, New York, N.Y. 10011
> Serves as clearing house of information about blindness; promotes the development of educational and other services for the blind; prints book in Braille, large type, and manufactures talking books.

National Industries for the Blind, Inc., 50 West 44th Street, New York, N.Y. 10036
> Serves as a central agency in assisting local agencies to develop work programs to provide permanent, paid employment for the

blind. Helps develop new products for manufacture by the blind, and cooperates to prevent exploitation of blind workers.

National Society for the Prevention of Blindness, Inc., 16 East 40th Street, New York, N.Y. 10016

Provides information designed to assist in developing programs to prevent blindness. Supports eye research, cooperates in educational programs, eye examinations, glaucoma detection. Also promotes educational facilities for partially sighted, and provides information on low vision aids and clinics.

Medical and Research Organizations

Eye-Bank Association of America, 2041 Queen Street, Winston-Salem, North Carolina 27103

Collects and furnishes corneas, scleras, and vitreous without charge to patients throughout the United States.

Fight for Sight, Inc., National Council to Combat Blindness, Inc., 41 West 57th Street, New York, N.Y. 10019

Supports and finances eye research in medical schools, hospitals, and eye centers, also serves as information center regarding needs of eye research.

Research to Prevent Blindness, Inc., 598 Madison Avenue, New York, N.Y. 10022

Stimulates and supports basic research into causes and prevention of blinding eye diseases. Provides research grants to medical schools and other research centers.

Guide Dog Schools

Guide Dogs for the Blind, Inc., P.O. Box 1200, San Rafael, California 94902. (Serves states west of the Mississippi River.)

International Guiding Eyes, Inc., 5431 Denny Avenue, North Hollywood, California 91603

Leader Dogs for the Blind, 1039 South Rochester Road, Rochester, Michigan 48063

The Seeing Eye, Inc., P.O. Box 375, Morristown, New Jersey 07960

APPENDIX

Guide Dog Foundation for the Blind, Inc., 109–19 72nd Avenue, Forest Hills, New York 11375

Guiding Eyes for the Blind, Inc., 106 East 41st Street, New York, N.Y. 10017

Pilot Dogs, Inc., 625 West Town Street, Columbus, Ohio 43215

Organizations Providing Reading and Educational Materials

American Printing House for the Blind, Inc., 1839 Frankfort Avenue, Louisville, Kentucky 40206
> Prints books, magazines, music in Braille; produces talking books, recorded tapes, large-type books; manufactures educational aids for the blind.

Braille Institute of America, Inc., 741 North Vermont Avenue, Los Angeles, California 90029
> Prints books and periodicals in both Braille and Moon type.

Clovernook Printing House for the Blind, 7000 Hamilton Avenue, Cincinnati, Ohio 45231
> Prints books, magazines, catalogues and other materials in Braille for such national organizations as the Library of Congress, American Legion, Lions International, American Foundation for the Blind.

Hadley School for the Blind, 700 Elm Street, Winnetka, Illinois 60093
> Offers correspondence school courses in academic or vocational subjects. Textbooks along with lesson by lesson tutorial service offered in Braille, and/or on records or tape. No charge for courses.

Howe Press of Perkins School for the Blind, 175 North Beacon Street, Watertown, Massachusetts 02172
> Prints Braille books, maps, music, mathematical aids, etc.

Jewish Braille Institute of America, Inc., 48 East 74th Street, New York, N.Y. 10021
> Publishes Braille prayer books in Hebrew and English, talking

books in Hebrew, Yiddish, and English. Records elementary and high school textbooks.

John Milton Society for the Blind, 475 Riverside Drive, New York, N.Y. 10027

An agency of the Protestant churches of the United States and Canada, it publishes free religious literature, periodicals, prayer and hymn books in Braille, also produces talking books.

Music for the Blind, Inc., 330 West 72nd Street, New York, N.Y. 10023

Publishes *The Braille Musician,* arranges professional discussions and musical programs.

Recording for the Blind, Inc., 215 East 58th Street, New York, N.Y. 10022

Produces and provides free on loan records and tapes of textbooks and other educational materials. Over 12,000 titles in every field of study listed in current catalogue (available on request).

Volunteers Service for the Blind, Inc., 332 South 13th Street, Philadelphia, Pennsylvania 19107

Provides Braille and sound recordings on record or tape of books and periodicals. Also provides reading services for blind students, professional and business people.

Xavier Society for the Blind, 154 East 23rd Street, New York, N.Y. 10010

National Catholic publishing house and library for the blind. Publishes religious books in Braille and talking book form; maintains free circulating library of Braille books and talking books.

Organizations Having Special Interest in Service to the Blind

Association of Junior Leagues of America, Inc., c/o Waldorf-Astoria, 301 Park Avenue, New York, N.Y. 10022

Provides trained volunteers to work with organizations serving

APPENDIX

the blind in educational projects, rehabilitation, and prevention of blindness.

Delta Gamma Foundation, 3250 Riverside Drive, Columbus, Ohio 43221

Promotes local community service by members, maintains scholarship program for teachers of blind and for partially seeing children.

Lions International, 209 North Michigan Avenue, Chicago, Illinois 60601

Engaged in wide range of activities for the blind, promoting legislation, furnishing guide dogs, distributing Braille literature and blind aids, developing educational and job training programs, setting blind people up in business.

National Federation of the Blind, Inc., 2652 Shasta Road, Berkeley, California 94708

Federation of organizations of blind people, studies and promotes legislation to improve social and economic conditions for the blind; grants scholarships to blind students to study law, medicine, engineering, architecture and natural sciences.

For complete listing of agencies and organizations see: *Directory of Agencies Serving Blind Persons in the United States,* published by the American Foundation for the Blind, Inc., 15 West 16th Street, New York, N.Y. 10011

Bibliography

Atkinson, D. T. *Magic, Myth and Medicine.* New York: World, 1956.
Bernal, J. D. *Science in History.* New York: Cameron Associates, 1957.
Best, C. H., and N. B. Taylor. *Physiological Basis of Medical Practice.* Baltimore: Williams & Wilkins, 1950.
Best, C. H., and N. B. Taylor. *The Human Body.* New York: Holt, 1956.
Browne, E. G. *Arabian Medicine.* Cambridge: Cambridge University Press, 1921.
Castiglioni, Arturo. *A History of Medicine,* ed. E. B. Krumbhaar. New York: Knopf, 1958.

BIBLIOGRAPHY

Chusid, J. G., and J. J. McDonald. *Correlative Neuroanatomy and Functional Neurology.* Los Altos, California: Lange Medical Publications, 1962.

Ciba Foundation Symposium. *Medicine in Ancient Egypt.* Vol. I, No. 10, Jan. 1940.

Dampier, W. C. *A History of Science.* Cambridge: Cambridge University Press, 1949.

Davson, Hugh. *The Physiology of the Eye.* Boston: Little, Brown, 1963.

Duke-Elder, W. S. *Textbook of Ophthalmology.* London: Kimpton, 1932.

Ebbell, B., trans. *The Papyrus Ebers.* London: Milford, 1937.

Frazer, J. G. *The Golden Bough.* London: Macmillan, 1910.

Granit, Ragnar. *Sensory Mechanisms of the Retina.* Oxford: Oxford University Press, 1947.

Helmholtz, H. von. *Treatise on Physiological Optics.* New York: Dover, 1924.

Luria, A. R. *Higher Cortical Functions in Man.* Trans. Basil Haigh. New York: Basic Books, 1965.

Polyak, S. L. *The Retina.* Chicago: University of Chicago Press, 1941.

Poynter, F. N. L., ed. *The Brain and Its Functions.* Oxford: Blackwell, 1958.

Randolph, Vance. *Ozark Superstitions.* New York: Dover, 1947.

Rawdon-Smith, A. F. *Theories of Sensation.* Cambridge: Cambridge University Press, 1938.

Turnley, Joseph. *The Language of the Eye.* London: Partridge, 1856.

Wolff, Eugene. *Anatomy of the Eye and Orbit.* Philadelphia: Saunders, 1961.

Wright, W. D. *Researches on Normal and Defective Color Vision.* London: Kimpton, 1946.

Glossary

accommodation: the ability of the eye to adjust for varying distances
acetylcholine: a chemical compound essential for the transmission of nerve impulses
albinism, ocular: complete absence of pigment in the eyes
amaurosis: blindness occurring without any apparent lesion of the eye
amblyopia: impairment of vision with no detectable organic lesion
aneurysm: a sac formed by the dilation of the walls of an artery or vein, and filled with blood
angiitis: inflammation of a blood vessel
angle of anterior chamber: junction between iris and cornea through which the aqueous flows

GLOSSARY

angoid streaks: bands appearing in the retina, often associated with systemic disease

aniridia: absence of the iris

anisekonia: a condition in which the image of an object seen by one eye differs in size and shape from that seen by the other eye

anisometropia: a difference in the refractive power of each eye, resulting in a difference in the apparent size of objects seen

antibody: part of defense mechanism against disease

antigen: substance which induces formation of antibodies

aphakia: having no lens in the eye, e.g., after cataract removal

aqueous humor: fluid in the anterior chamber of the eye

arcus senilis: a white ring around the margin of the cornea, especially in the aged

asthenopia: weakness or tiring of the eyes, dimness of vision

astigmatism: visual defect caused by abnormal curvature of the cornea

atropine: drug that paralyzes parasympathetic nerve action; applied locally to the eye to dilate the pupil and paralyze ciliary muscle

autoimmunity: allergy to one's own tissue

blepharitis: inflammation of the eyelids

blepharospasm: spasm of eyelid muscles

blind spot: normal defect in visual field due to position at which optic nerve enters the eye

buphthalmos: enlargement of the eye

canaliculus (lacrimal): narrow tubular passage, tear duct

canthus: the angle at either end of the slit between the eyelids

cataract: an opacity of the lens

    incipient: any cataract in its early stages, or one which has sectors of opacity with clear spaces intervening

    mature: a cataract in which the lens is completely opaque and ready for operation

    hypermature: a cataract in which the lens has become either solid and shrunken, or soft and liquid

    congenital: a cataract that originates before birth

    senile: a hard opacity of the lens in the aging eye

    traumatic: cataract following an injury

choked disc: swelling of the optic nerve
chorioretinitis: inflammation of the choroid and retina
choroid: vascular layer of the eyes, the function of which is to nourish the retina
ciliary body: portion of vascular layer of eye whose function is secretion of aqueous humor
coloboma: a congenital defect in which a portion of a structure of the eye is absent
cone, retinal: a specialized visual cell in the retina, responsible for sharpness of vision and color vision
conical cornea, keratoconus: a conical protrusion of the cornea
conjunctiva: the delicate membrane that lines the eyelids and covers the exposed surface of the eyeball
contact lens, corneal: contact lens molded to the cornea
contact lens, scleral: contact lens molded to the sclera
corticosteroids: cortisone derivatives
cryosurgery: use of low temperature in surgery
cup, optic: depression in the center of the optic disc
cyclitis: inflammation of the ciliary body
cycloplegia: paralysis of the ciliary muscle
cytomegalic inclusion disease: retinal viral inflammation
dacryocystitis: inflammation of the lacrimal sac
detachment of retina: a condition in which the inner layers of the retina are separated from the pigment layer
diopter: a unit designating the refractive power of a lens
diplopia: double vision
disc, optic: the optic nerve within the eye
electroretinogram: a record of changes of electrical potential in the retina after stimulation by light
emmetropia: perfect vision
endophthalmitis: inflammation of the interior structures of the eye
enucleation: surgical removal of the eye
esotropia: actual deviation of the visual axis of one eye toward the other; "crossed eyes"
esphoria: a tendency to deviation of the visual axis of one eye toward the other

GLOSSARY

exophoria: a tendency to deviation of the axis of one eye away from the other

exophthalmos: abnormal protrusion of the eyeball

exotropia: actual deviation of the axis of one eye away from the other; "walleyes"

flash blindness: loss of vision resulting from intense light, such as that of an atomic blast

fovea centralis: a tiny depression in the center of the macula, the area of greatest visual acuity

fundus: the base or remote interior of an organ such as the eye

glaucoma: a condition of the eye characterized by increased intraocular pressure

> *acute, closed angle:* glaucoma caused by obstruction of the filtration angle by the base of the iris
>
> *chronic simple, open angle:* glaucoma in which the angle of the anterior chamber is open and free from obstruction
>
> *congenital:* glaucoma present at birth due to a defect in the angle of the anterior chamber
>
> *absolute:* a final stage in which vision is completely and permanently lost

gonioscopy: examination of the anterior chamber of the eye

gonorrheal ophthalmia: blinding eye disease of newborn infants acquired in the birth canal

hemianopia: defective vision or blindness in half of the visual field

herpes simplex: an acute virus disease marked by groups of watery blisters on the skin and mucous membranes; the most common cause of blindness due to a corneal disease

histoplasmosis: parasitic inflammation affecting the eye

hyperopia: farsightedness

hyphaema: hemorrhage into the anterior chamber of the eye

intraocular pressure: the pressure of the fluid within the eye

iridectomy: surgical removal of part of the iris

iridocyclitis: inflammation of the iris and the ciliary body

iritis: inflammation of the iris

keratitis: inflammation of the cornea, usually characterized by loss of transparency, and dullness

keratoconus: conical cornea, a conical protrusion of the cornea

keratoprosthesis: corneal implant, usually of plastic material; artificial cornea

lacrimal: (adj.), pertaining to the tears, or to the structure conducting or secreting tears

lagophthalmos: a condition in which the eye cannot be completely closed

lens: lens of the eye: a transparent biconvex body, situated between the posterior chamber and the vitreous, through which the light rays are focused on the retina

lenticular: (adj.), pertaining to or shaped like a lens

leukoma: a dense white opacity of the cornea

levator muscle: muscle which raises the eyelid

limbus: a border; the edge of the cornea where it joins the sclera

macula lutea: an oval area in the center of the retina devoid of blood vessels

microphthalmos: a rare developmental defect in which the eyeballs are abnormally small

miosis: reduction in the size of the pupil

miotic: a drug which causes a reduction in the size of the pupil

muscae volitantes: small floating spots seen when looking at a bright uniform field, such as the sky; attributed to minute remnants of embryonic structure in the vitreous humor

mydriasis: increase in pupil size

myopia: nearsightedness

myopic degeneration: a form of nearsightedness which may lead to blindness

needling (of cataract): a surgical procedure in which the lens is punctured to allow the absorption of the lens substance

neuritis, optic: inflammation of a nerve, e.g., the optic nerve

    retrobulbar: inflammation of the orbital portion of the optic nerve

nystagmus: a regular, rapid, characteristically involuntary movement or rotation of the eye

oculist: ophthalmologist (still used in England)

oculomotor: (adj.), pertaining to the movement of the eye

GLOSSARY

opacity: the condition of being opaque
ophthalmodynamometer: an instrument for measuring the blood pressure in the retinal artery
ophthalmologist: a medical practitioner specializing in the medical and surgical care of the eyes
ophthalmoscopy, direct: the mirrored observation of an upright image of the interior of the eye
ophthalmoscopy, indirect: the observation of an inverted image of the interior of the eye
optic atrophy: degeneration of the optic nerve fibers; visual loss usually accompanies this condition
optic chiasm: an arrangement of nerve fibers in which the optic nerves of both eyes cross at a junction near the pituitary gland
optic disc: the portion of the optic nerve within the eye which is formed by the meeting of all the retinal nerve fibers at the level of the retina
optic neuritis: inflammation of the optic nerve
optician: one who designs or manufactures optical instruments, glasses
optometrist: an expert in optometry; nonmedical visual care
orbicularis: an eyelid muscle which closes the eye
orbit: the cavity in the skull which contains the eyeball
orthoptics: the teaching and training process for the elimination of strabismus
pallor of disc: paleness of the optic nerve, suggesting atrophy
palpebral: pertaining to the eyelid
panophthalmitis: inflammation of all the structures of the eye
papilledema: noninflammatory edema of the optic nerve head
pathway, visual: the neural path of visual impulses
pemphigus: a progressive and often fatal condition of blistering and scarring of the mucous membranes and the skin which can affect the eye
perimeter: an instrument for measuring the field of vision
phakoma: a small grayish white tumor in the retina
phlyctenule: a minute ulcerated nodule of the cornea or conjunctiva
phoria: a tendency to deviation of the eyes from normal
photophobia: abnormal sensitivity to and discomfort from light

phthisis bulbi: shrinking, wasting, and atrophy of the eyeball
pigment epithelium: a layer of cells in the retina containing pigment granules
pilocarpine: a substance that causes the pupil to contract
pituitary ablation: destruction of pituitary gland
pleoptics: a technique of eye exercises designed to develop fuller vision and binocular cooperation
posterior pole of eye: the center of the posterior curvature of the eye
presbyopia: impairment of vision due to advancing years or old age
pterygium: a growth of the conjunctiva considered to be due to a degenerative process caused by long-continued irritation as from exposure to wind and dust
ptosis: a paralytic drooping of the upper eyelid
pupil: the opening at the center of the iris of the eye for the transmission of light
rectus muscle: a muscle attached to the eyeball which controls eye movements
reflex, corneal: blinking or winking in response to tactile stimulation of the cornea; reflection of light from the cornea
reflex, pupillary: constriction of the pupil when stimulated by light
refractive error: a defect in the eye that prevents light waves from being brought to a single focus exactly on the retina
retina: the innermost of the three tunics of the eyeball, surrounding the vitreous body and continuous posteriorly with the optic nerve
retinal hole: a space where the retina has pulled away from the underlying choroid tissue
retinitis pigmentosa: a hereditary degeneration and atrophy of the retina
retinoblastoma: a tumor arising from retinal germ cells
retino-choroiditis: inflammation of the retina and the choroid
retinopathy: a disease of the retina due to various causes
    diabetic: changes in the retina due to diabetes mellitus
    hypertensive: a disease of the retina associated with essential or malignant hypertension

GLOSSARY

retinoscope: an instrument for measuring the refractive state of the eye

retrobulbar: situated or occurring behind the eyeball

retrolental fibroplasia: a disease of the retina in which a mass of scar tissue forms in back of the lens; associated with premature birth and oxygen inhalation

rubeosis iridis: condition characterized by a new formation of vessels and connective tissue on the surface of the eye

sac, conjunctival: the potential space, lined by conjunctiva, between the eyelids and the eyeball

sac, lacrimal: the dilated upper end of the nasolacrimal canal

Schlemm's canal: a circular channel at the junction of the sclera and cornea through which aqueous humor leaves the eye

sclera: the tough, white, protective coat of the eye

scotoma: a blind or partially blind area in the visual field

separation of retina: separation of the retina from its pigment epithelium layer

slit-lamp: an instrument producing a slender beam of light for illuminating any reasonably transparent structure, as the cornea

spasm, lid (blepharospasm): a sudden, violent, involuntary contraction of the eyelid, attended by pain

squint, accommodative: that which is due to excessive or deficient accommodative effort

  convergent: that in which the visual axes converge; cross-eyed

  divergent: that in which the visual axes diverge

  paralytic: due to paralysis of an eye muscle

staphyloma: protrusion of the cornea or sclera resulting from inflammation

stereopsis: visual perception of depth or three-dimensional space

stereotactic surgery: use of three-dimensional localization in surgery

strabismus: squint; failure of the two eyes simultaneously to direct their gaze at the same object because of muscle imbalance

sty (hordeolum): inflammation of one or more of the sebaceous glands of the eyelids

subluxation: incomplete dislocation of the lens

GLOSSARY

sympathetic ophthalmia: inflammation of one eye due to an injury in the other eye

syndrome: a set of symptoms which occur together; a symptom complex

synechia: adhesions, usually of the iris to the cornea or lens

tarsal plate: the framework of connective tissue which gives shape to the eyelid

tarsorrhaphy: surgical attachment of upper and lower lids

tear film: microscopic film which constantly bathes cornea

Tenon's capsule: the fibrous membrane surrounding the sclera

tonography: the recording of changes in intraocular pressure produced by the constant application of a known weight on the globe of the eye

tonometer: an instrument for measuring the pressure inside the eye

trachoma: a chronic, contagious, viral infection of the conjunctiva and the cornea

tumbling: technique of removing cataract

ulcer, corneal: pathologic loss of substance of the surface of the cornea, due to progressive erosion and death of the tissues

uniocular: (adj.), pertaining to or affecting one eye

uveitis: inflammation of the vascular coat of the eye (choroid, ciliary body and the iris)

vision, central: vision elicited by stimuli impinging directly on the macula

vision, distant: vision for objects at a distance (usually from twenty feet or six meters)

vision, near: vision for objects at a distance corresponding to normal reading distance (thirteen to sixteen inches)

vision, peripheral: vision elicited by stimuli falling on areas of the retina distant from the macula

vision, photopic: vision attributed to cone function, characterized by the ability to discriminate colors and small detail; daylight vision

vision, scotopic: vision attributed to rod function, characterized by the lack of ability to discriminate colors and small detail, and effective primarily in the detection of movement and low luminous intensities

GLOSSARY

visual acuity: ability of the eye to perceive the shape of objects in the direct line of vision, sharpness of sight

visual axis: the line of gaze, a straight line from the object seen, through the center of the pupil to the macula lutea

visual cortex: final station of visual impulses in the brain; sensory area of brain responsible for vision

visual field: the area of physical space visible to an eye in a given position

vitreous, or vitreous body: transparent, colorless mass of soft gelatinous material filling the eyeball behind the lens

water drinking test: provocative test for glaucoma; the patient drinks one quart of water after fasting, and the intraocular pressure is measured every fifteen minutes

xerophthalmia: conjunctivitis with atrophy and no liquid discharge; produces a dry, lusterless condition of the eyeball

zonule of Zinn: the suspensory apparatus of the lens

Index

ABERRATION, 59–60
accommodation, 39
acuity, visual, 11, 13, 81–82, 186; and strabismus, 74, 75; and amblyopia, 77
age: and eye, 12–13, 39, 57, 59, 67–71; and peripheral vision, 42; and senile cataract, 91–92; and detached retina, 99, 100; and macular degeneration, 106
agencies, for the blind, 178–179, 219–224
alcohol: and peripheral vision, 42, 80; and color blindness, 44; and exotropia, 73; and "seeing double," 77–80; and toxic amblyopia, 122
allergy, 124, 127, 146–148; to drugs, 209; *see also* autoimmunity
alpha chymotrypsin, 96
amauroscope, 215–216
amblyopia, 61, 74–77, 122, 164, 211–213
aneurysms, 107–108, 109
aniseikonia, 191–192
anisometropia, 76
aqueous humor, 37; and glaucoma,

INDEX

82–83, 86, 88; and cataracts, 204
arterioles, 111
astigmatism, 36, 60, 66, 70, 186; corrective lenses for, 189, 194; and heredity, 209
atherosclerosis, 108–109, 110–111, 143
Atromid-S, 110–111, 112
atrophy, optic, 122
autoimmunity, 116, 118, 145–146, 202

BANGERTER, DR. ALFRED, 77
Beadle, George W., 210
bifocal lenses. *See* lenses, corrective
binocular fusion. *See* fusion
black eye, 153–154
blepharoconjunctivitis, contact, 147–148
blind spot, 42–43, 60, 121
blind zone, 42
blindness, 3–4, 175–182; causes of, 62–63, 201; night, 142, 209; rubella-instigated, 144–145; as result of injury, 151–153; ancient concept of, 176–177; legal definition in U.S., 177
books for the blind, 180–182
Bradley, Dr. R. F., 109
Braille, 176, 178, 179–181
Braille, Louis, 180
brain, 5, 6, 23, 27; and recognition, 46–50; and relative distance, 50–52; and optical illusions, 52–53; and image inhibition, 73, 74
Breinin, Dr. Goodwin M., 77
burns, 154–155

CAMERA, compared to eye, 25, 27, 57, 213; light-regulating system, 37–38; and distance accommodation, 68

Campo, Dr. Armando del, 215–216
Canal of Schlemm, 82, 85
cancer, 137–138, 160
cannulation-perfusion, 208
Carrod, Sir Archibald E., 210
Castroviejo, Ramón, 130
cataracts, 20–21, 39, 61, 71, 89–96, 99, 115, 201, 206; infantile, 76; surgery for, 21, 89–90, 93–96; symptoms of, 91, 157–158; congenital, 92; traumatic, 92; secondary, 92; metabolic, 92, 107; treatment of, 93–97; and uveitis, 116; from sunlight, 160; prevention, 203–205; genetic component in, 209, 210
chemotherapy, 138
children: strabismus in, 73–75; amblyopia in, 77; uveitis in, 114–115; and eye protection, 163–168; and "seeing habits," 168–172; *see also* infants
choroid, 36, 206; and detached retina, 62, 98–99, 100; in uveal tract, 113; melanoma of, 138
chromosomes and mongolism, 210–211
ciliary body, 36, 38, 68–69, 71; and glaucoma, 82, 86; in uveal tract, 113
Clark, Dr. W. Bruce, 214–215
Cogan, Dr. David, 108
color, 11–12, 43–45; and cones, 39, 43–44; and optical illusions, 52–53
color blindness, 44–45, 62, 209
cones, 39–40, 42, 43–44
conjunctiva, 28, 123–126, 128
conjunctivitis, 62, 123–124, 147
contact lenses, 97, 130, 192, 193–200, 203, 204–205; pros and cons, 194–196, 199; scleral, 194, 197–198; flush-fitting scleral, 194,

INDEX

198–199, 200; corneal, 194, 196–197; *see also* lenses, corrective
cornea, 28, 36, 37, 127–130; transplant of, 128, 130–135; artificial, 205–206
corneal lenses. *See* contact lenses
cortex, 48–50
cortisone, 114, 118, 124; *see also* drugs; steroids
crossed eyes. *See* esotropia
crystalline lens, 11, 37, 38–39, 65; and aging process, 68–69; cataractous, 91, 93; *see also* lenses, corrective
Cüppers, Dr. Kurt, 77

DACRYOCYSTITIS, 139
dacryostenosis, 139
depth perception, 41, 51, 74
Descartes, René, 24–25, 27
detached retina, 61–62, 92, 98–105, 119
DeVoe, Dr. Arthur Gerard, 128, 206
diabetes, 59, 71, 142, 207; and retinal damage, 62, 106–111; and sugar cataracts, 92, 203; and fat metabolism, 108; and genetic susceptibility, 210
diazoxide, 112
diplopia, 73–74, 165–166
disease, ocular, 201–203, 206–208; *see also under specific disease*
dogs, guide, for the blind, 179
double image. *See* diplopia
drugs, 202; and glaucoma, 86, 88, 206–207; and cataracts, 92–93; and diabetic retinopathy, 110–111, 207; sulfonamide, 125; adverse effects of, 208–209
Duke-Elder, Dr. W. S., 99

EBERS PAPYRUS, 19, 20, 125
Egypt, 16, 18–21, 183, 201

emmetropia, 60
enzymes, 96, 210–211
episcleritis, 135
erysipelas, 127
esotropia, 60, 72–75, 80, 164
evil eye. *See* superstition
exophthalmos, 140, 142
exotropia, 60, 73, 80
eye, human: other forms of, 4, 6–8; evolution of, 9–13; and superstition, 14–17; earliest studies of, 18–25; artificial, 20; structure of, 26–37; and light regulation, 37–38; vulnerability of, 57; structural abnormalities, 59; deviated, 75; hazards to exterior of, 123–136; sensitivity of, 141–144; first aid for, 151–153; fatigue and, 155; in children, 163–172; research on, 206–208
eye banks, 130–135
eyeball, 60; mobility of, 40–41, 190–191, 192; in myopia, 64–65; in hyperopia, 65; protrusion of, 140, 142
eyelid, 10, 28, 126–127

FAGER, DR. C. A., 109
farsightedness. *See* hyperopia
Feree, Dr. John W., 163, 164
Fialkow, Dr. P. J., 44
Filatov, V. P., 130
Finnerty, Dr. Frank, 112
floaters, 100, 120
florescein, 207, 208
fovea, 11, 25; centralis, 40, 187; in infants, 73; in amblyopia, 77
fundus, optic, 143
fusion, 41; binocular, 73, 80; and anisometropia, 76

GALACTOSEMIA, 203, 211
German measles, 144–145
Girard, Dr. Louis J., 197, 198–199

239

INDEX

glasses. See lenses, corrective
glaucoma, 37, 61, 71, 81–88, 99, 115, 145; symptoms of, 83–84, 158; test for, 85–86; treatment of, 86–88, 90–91; and secondary cataract, 92; detection of, 206–207; heredity and, 209
Gonin, Jules, 104–105
goniscope, 84–85
gout, 59, 145–146
Graefe, Albrecht von, 88, 96
Gregg, Sir Norman McAlister, 144

HALLUCINATION, 47; see also optical illusion
Helmholtz, Hermann von, 85, 88
hemorrhage, 126, 142, 143
heredity, and sight, 45, 60, 202, 209–211
herpes zoster ophthalmicus, 127
histoplasma capsulatum, 115
hordeolum. See sty
hormones, 108, 110
Hubel, Dr. David, 212
hyperopia, 60, 65, 70, 185, 186; corrective lenses for, 188–189; and heredity, 209
hypertension, 59, 62, 71; retinopathy of, 111–112, 143, 207
hypertropia, 60
hypophysectomy, 109, 110
hypotropia, 60

INFANTS: vision in, 73; cataracts in, 76, 144; and rubella, 144–145; galactosemia and PKU in, 211; see also children
infections, 62, 71, 128, 208
infectious eczematoid dermatitis, 148
inflammation, 62, 145–146; see also uveitis
injury, 151–155, 168–169

iridacyclitis, 114
iridectomy, 88, 96
iris, 11, 36–38, 69, 96, 113, 145

JAEGER, E., 186
Jepson, Dr. C. Neal, 109

KAUFMAN, DR. HERBERT E., 135
Keller, Helen, 177
Kepler, Johannes, 24
keratitis, 128
kidney disease, 62, 71, 142
Kinoshita, Dr. Jin, 204
Kinsey, Dr. V. Everett, 92, 204
Kuwabara, Dr. Toichiro, 108

LACRIMAL GLANDS, 28; see also tears
Laqueur, Louis, 88
laser, 105
Lederberg, Joshua, 210
lenses, corrective, 12, 23, 39, 58–59, 60, 65–66, 188–192; for reading, 70; bifocal, 70–71, 189–191; and deviated eye, 75; and cataracts, 97, 194–195; and safety, 159; historical background of, 183–185; testing for, 185–187, 202; trifocal, 191; see also crystalline lenses; contact lenses
light, 5–8, 27, 37; artificial, 161–162
liver disease, 44, 62, 71
lysozyme, 28

MCDONALD, DR. P. ROBB, 99–100, 104
McLean, Dr. John M., 96–97
macula lutea, 40, 83, 186–187
magnifying glass, 23, 183, 184
Maumenee, Dr. A. Edward, 114, 115
Maxwell, James Clerk, 6

microphthalmos, 145
Milton, John, 177
miotics, 86, 88
mirror vision, 165
mongolism, 210–211
Muller, F. A., 198
multiple sclerosis, 142
musical scores, for the blind, 180
myopia, 60, 64, 70, 186; and retinal detachment, 99; corrective lenses for, 188, 189–190; and heredity, 209

NEARSIGHTEDNESS. See myopia
neuritis, optic. See papillitis
Noorden, Dr. Gunter K. von, 75, 164, 212
nutrition, and the eye, 71, 142

OCCLUSION THERAPY, 75, 77
O'Connor, Dr. G. Richard, 147
oculist, defined, 58
ophthalmia, 19, 147
ophthalmologist, 58, 70, 186
ophthalmology, science of, 58
ophthalmoscope, 85
optic nerve, 119–122; disorders of, 120–122
optic neuritis. See papillitis
optical illusion, 52–53
optician, 58–59, 186
optics, science of, 58
optometrist, 58, 70, 186
orbit, 27–28, 40–41, 139–140
orbital lymphoma, 138

PAPILLEDEMA, 120–121
papillitis, 62, 121, 140, 142
Patz, Dr. Arnall, 107
Penfield, Dr. Wilder, 47
periodicals, for the blind, 180–181
periosteum, 28
phenylketonuria (PKU), 211

photocoagulation, 105, 109
photosensitivity, 7–9
Pierce, Dr. L. H., 99
pink eye. See conjunctivitis
pleoptic therapy, 77
publishers, for the blind, 181–182
presbyopia, 60, 69–71, 186; corrective lenses for, 189, 190
pupil, 11, 37–38, 69

RADIATION, 138
recognition, role of brain in, 46–53; and perception, 213–215
Reddy, Dr. D. V. N., 204
Reese, Dr. Algernon, 137–138
Reese, Dr. S. B., 109
refraction, tests for, 187
refractive error. See aberration
rehabilitation, optical, 96–97
retina, 5, 10–11, 36, 37, 38, 39–40; stimulation of, 76, 212–215; and diabetes, 142; see also detached retina
retinitis, 62
retinoblastoma, 137–138
retinopathy, 62, 206; diabetic, 106–111, 142, 143, 207; hypertensive, 106, 111–112, 142, 143, 207
retinoscope, 187
rhabdomyosarcoma, 137
rheumatoid arthritis, 114, 116, 135–136, 145–146
rods, 39–40, 42
rubella, 144–145

SABIN, DR. ALBERT B., 125
Scheie, Dr. Harold, 84
Schiotz, Hjalmar, 88
sclera, 36, 127, 128, 135–136
scleral lenses. See contact lenses
scleritis, 135–136
sight, 44–45; development of, 7-13; three-dimensional, 41–43;

INDEX

problems of, 57–63; eyeless, 215–216; *see also* vision
Smith, Priestly, 88
Smith, Dr. R. T., 99
smoking, effect on vision, 42, 44, 122
Snellen, Herman, 186; eye-chart tests, 58, 165, 186
squint, accommodative, 61; *see also* strabismus
staphyloma, 136
steroids, 114, 118; and optic neuritis, 121; and conjunctivitis, 124; hazards of, 206–207; *see also* drugs
Straatsma, Dr. Bradley R., 145
strabismus, 60–61, 72–75, 164; treatment for, 74–75; in mongolism, 210
sty, 126
sun, hazards from, 160–162
superstition, and the eye, 14–17, 93
surgery, 93–94, 202; ancient, 20; for esotropia, 75; and glaucoma, 86, 88; and cataract, 93–96; to reattach retina, 104–105
survival, and sight, 4–5, 6, 12

"TALKING BOOKS," 176, 180–181
Tatum, Edward L., 210
tears, 28, 138–139; and contact lenses, 198
Templeton, Alec, 177
thermocautery, 104–105
Thomas, Tudor, 130
Thygeson, Dr. P., 125
thyroid gland, 140, 142
tonometer, 85, 88
toxocara canis, 115

toxoplasma gondi, 115
trabecula, 82, 88
trachoma, 124–125
transplants, corneal. *See* cornea
tumors, 137–138, 206, 207–208; *see also* cancer
Tuohy, Kevin, 193
Turnley, Joseph, *The Language of the Eye*, 17

ULCER, corneal, 199
uvea, 36
uveitis, 62, 113–118, 206, 208; causes of, 114–116; treatment of, 116–118

VASCULAR DISEASE, 109
vision, 41–43; peripheral, 41–42, 80, 84; normal, 58–59; and genetic susceptibility, 210; stimulation of, 211–215, *see also* sight
visual acuity. *See* acuity, visual
visual association areas, 49
vitreous humor, 37; and detached retina, 100, 104, 105, 119; and the optic nerve, 119–122
vitreous opacities, 100, 120

WETZIG, DR. PAUL C., 109
Whately, George, 190
Wiesel, Dr. Torsten, 212
World Health Organization, 124

XEROX, 182
xylose, 204

YALE UNIVERSITY, 42, 77–80

ZUSCHLAG, DR. HANS GERT, 80

RE51

**NO LONGER THE PROPERTY
OF THE
UNIVERSITY OF R.I. LIBRARY**

3 1222 00118 1109

DATE DUE		
~~MAY 23 1982~~		
~~MAY 13 1983~~		
NOV 02 1983		
APR 04 1984	MAY 17 1992	
DEC 10 1984	DEC 08 1992	
	DEC 01 1995	
NOV 18 1985		
APR 16 1986	DEC 10 2002	
SEP 12 1989		
NOV 10 1992		

GAYLORD   PRINTED IN U.S.A.